An archaeology of lunacy

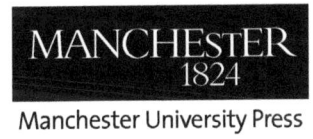
Manchester University Press

Social Archaeology and Material Worlds

Series editors
Joshua Pollard and Duncan Sayer

Social Archaeology and Material Worlds aims to forefront dynamic and cutting-edge social approaches to archaeology. It brings together volumes about past people, social and material relations and landscape as explored through an archaeological lens. Topics covered may include memory, performance, identity, gender, life course, communities, materiality, landscape and archaeological politics and ethnography. The temporal scope runs from prehistory to the recent past, while the series' geographical scope is global. Books in this series bring innovative, interpretive approaches to important social questions within archaeology. Interdisciplinary methods which use up-to-date science, history or both, in combination with good theoretical insight, are encouraged. The series aims to publish research monographs and well-focused edited volumes that explore dynamic and complex questions, the why, how and who of archaeological research.

Previously published

Neolithic cave burials: Agency, structure and environment
Rick Peterson

The Irish tower house: Society, economy and environment, c. 1300-1650
Victoria L. McAlister

Forthcoming

Images in the making: Art, process, archaeology
Ing-Marie Back Danielsson and Andrew Meirion Jones (eds)

Communities and knowledge production in archaeology
Julia Roberts, Kathleen Sheppard, Jonathan Trigg and Ulf Hansson (eds)

Early Anglo-Saxon cemeteries: Kinship, community and mortuary space
Duncan Sayer

Urban Zooarchaeology
James Morris

An archaeology of innovation: Approaching social and technological change in human society
Catherine J. Frieman

An archaeology of lunacy

Managing madness
in early nineteenth-century asylums

Katherine Fennelly

Manchester University Press

Copyright © Katherine Fennelly 2019

The right of Katherine Fennelly to be identified as the author of this work has been asserted by her in accordance with the Copyright, Designs and Patents Act 1988.

Published by Manchester University Press
Altrincham Street, Manchester M1 7JA, UK
www.manchesteruniversitypress.co.uk

British Library Cataloguing-in-Publication Data is available

ISBN 978 1 5261 2649 8 hardback

First published 2019

The publisher has no responsibility for the persistence or accuracy of URLs for any external or third-party internet websites referred to in this book, and does not guarantee that any content on such websites is, or will remain, accurate or appropriate.

Typeset by Servis Filmsetting Ltd, Stockport, Cheshire

This book is dedicated to my father, and in memory of my mother.

Contents

List of figures	*p.* viii
List of tables	x
Preface	xi
Acknowledgements	xv
Table of legislation	xvii
1 Introduction	1
2 Management	32
3 Administration	69
4 Movement	115
5 Conclusions	145
References	157
Index	173

Figures

1.1 Facade of St Patrick's Hospital, Dublin (c. 1890–1910), courtesy of the National Library of Ireland.   11

2.1 Richmond District Lunatic Asylum ground floor (1814). Line drawing by author, based on original plans by Francis Johnston (1814).   59

2.2 West Riding District Lunatic Asylum plans by Watson and Pritchett (1819). Line drawing by author, based on plans by Watson and Pritchett (1819).   62

2.3 Expenditure on food in two Irish asylums from 1844–51, spanning the peak years of the Great Famine (after The National Archives of the United Kingdom: Audits of Maryborough: AO 19/48/14; The National Archives of the United Kingdom: Audits of Richmond District Lunatic Asylum AO 19/48/17).   66

3.1 Carlow District Lunatic Asylum ground floor (1831). Line drawing by author, based on original plans by William Murray (1831).   76

3.2 Schematic for a cupola at Maryborough District Lunatic Asylum. Line drawing by author, based on William Murray's original schematic (1832).   77

3.3 Example of fork from the Maryborough District Lunatic Asylum, with asylum stamp. Private Collection, photograph by author.   90

3.4 Facade of administration block at St Fintan's Hospital, Portlaoise, formerly the Maryborough District Lunatic Asylum. Photograph by author.   92

3.5 Schematic for the lodge at Maryborough District Lunatic Asylum. Line drawing by author, based on William Murray's original schematic (1830).   103

3.6 Platter fragment with Maryborough District Asylum stamp. Private Collection, photograph by author. 110

4.1 Submitted designs for West Riding District Lunatic Asylum. Clockwise from top right: Bevans' radial plan; Hainton's U-shaped plan; Lindley, Woodhead and Hurst linear plan. Line drawings by author, based on original plans by James Bevans, Francis Hainton, and Lindley, Woodhead, and Hurst. 122

4.2 Access analyses of Richmond Lunatic Asylum, Maryborough District Asylum, and the West Riding District Asylum. 140

4.3 Plan of Dublin (Co Dublin), showing wards. Line drawing by author, based on map of Dublin 1835–36. 142

Tables

4.1 Samuel Tuke's specifications for the West Riding Asylum, compared with plan features.   124

Preface

In the popular imagination, the historic lunatic asylum was a dark, monolithic institution of social confinement. Locked behind thick, damp walls, the popular perception of the ailing patients – closely guarded behind locked doors by hard-faced matrons and sly, brutal keepers – dominates the popular memory of lunatic asylums. This legacy of the asylum, born out of a number of factors, some based in fact and some in fictional accounts of urban institutions and correlations between asylum architecture and that of the reformed nineteenth-century prison, has carried over into popular media and is pervasive. As such, the perception of all asylums as marginal, brutal places of human suffering is reflected in the ways in which asylum buildings are reused and redeveloped across the British Isles. This book aims to redress the history of the built and material environment of the lunatic asylum, identifying early nineteenth-century ideas on how the treatment of the mad informed the architecture and material culture of the early nineteenth-century asylum. Approaching the asylum and the built environment of mental health provision as archaeological artefacts and landscapes, this book will draw together archival source material, material culture, built heritage, and cartographic information.

The subject matter of the book necessitates a short note on terminology in order to clarify usage. The terminology used in this book is of its period and consistent with the primary source material for the subject. The buildings will be referred to as lunatic asylums or asylums throughout, allowing for changes in the names of the buildings as time went on; a building which continued in use as a facility for treating mental illness will be referred to as an asylum in relation to the early nineteenth century, and a hospital when discussing changes in the twentieth century. For example, the Maryborough District Lunatic Asylum, one of the buildings examined in detail in this book, will be referred to as an asylum in the 1830s, but as a hospital, Portlaoighse Mental Hospital, when discussing changes to the building in the 1930s. This change in nomenclature is necessary to maintain consistency with the primary source material referred to throughout. Similarly, words like 'insane', 'madness', 'lunatic', and 'mad' will be used frequently, as this is consistent with the language employed at the time in question. For the same reason, though asylums are frequently conflated with prisons and workhouses of the period, the word 'patient' will be used to refer to the denizens of the asylums, consistent with the sources.

Primary source material relating to lunatic asylums in the nineteenth century is reasonably prolific. As government-run, or -regulated, institutions, asylums generated a significant amount of administrative material, most of which is accessible in public record offices or private archives. The archaeology of the lunatic asylum, of insanity, and of institutions in general, is a growing subfield of historical archaeology. The volume of material and breadth of different approaches adopted by researchers to study these (sometimes problematic) buildings means that this book is a contribution to a much larger body of work. As such, the subject of this book is the buildings, their builders, and the staff who were responsible for running them. For a patient-focused archaeological approach to lunatic asylums, I invite the reader to look at the work of Susan Piddock, cited frequently in this book, and papers on the subject published in the *International Journal of Historical Archaeology*, *Historical Archaeology*, and *Post-Medieval Archaeology* journals. Focusing on the materiality of reform, administration, and control, this book looks primarily at the buildings and their constructors and workers, often the enforcers of the rules, and their approaches to the ever-changing material landscape of the early nineteenth-century asylum.

It is difficult to detach completely from a subject matter like mental health. Many scholarly approaches to the subject are inspired or informed by personal engagements with mental illness or mental hospitals, and this book is no exception. My approach has been stimulated and informed by my experiences with these buildings before I ever approached them as an archaeologist. I was attracted to this research topic due to my familiarity with a former district asylum in Ireland where I was employed as a clerical assistant while I was an undergraduate student, but I had been familiar with the building even before that. The hospital, still in operation, had employed both of my parents, two of my siblings, and several uncles before me. As such, I approached the topic as a former employee, with a cognisance of the importance of representing only what narratives I had access to through the material culture and sources available. My knowledge of the Irish health service, and familiarity with psychiatric nurses in particular, meant that my fieldwork has been facilitated and aided by many current and former staff members of Irish and English psychiatric hospitals. Indeed, it is through these contacts made in provincial hospitals, small community-run museums, and through academic networks, that I gained access to materials and records which were saved from destruction by the enthusiasm and insight of the interested public. Community networks are vital for the study of historic buildings, especially those with problematic and underrepresented histories, like lunatic asylums. Maintaining a link with at least one associated community means that their voices and opinions on the direction of the research are heard and taken into consideration. This is key to maintaining relevance to these communities, who have been instrumental in building up historical networks of staff and even contributing to the development of residential neighbourhoods around institutions.

As well as the Maryborough Asylum, several other detailed case studies are referred to throughout, representing major changes at a national level and local practice at asylum level. Another asylum looked at in detail will be one I have lived in close proximity to while writing this book, the Lincoln City Asylum. Lincoln City Asylum was a pioneer of the non-restraint movement in asylum management and was one of two lunatic asylums in operation in the city of Lincoln in England at the end of the nineteenth century. The other asylum, located to the south of the city at Bracebridge Heath, represents an archetypical Victorian lunatic asylum, and the village which grew up around that institution signifies the historical importance of these buildings as services, employers, suppliers, and customers. Both the former Lincoln City Asylum and the Bracebridge Heath Asylum have undergone redevelopment in the 2010s, the former into a small-scale industrial complex and hotel and the latter into a domestic estate. These developments are just two of the purposes to which former asylum buildings are being put, with others in the planning process. As archaeologists, both academic and commercial, we are in a key position to inform on the impact these buildings have had on their locales, from early nineteenth-century origins as pioneers of what became psychological medicine, to later twentieth-century proving grounds for psychiatry, for better or worse. Far from marginal, these places occupy significant positions in local memory and beyond. Many of the key battles in psychiatry were fought in the draughty corridors and echoing verandas of these experimental building types. As employers, asylums consistently employed women on a meaningful scale from the early nineteenth century, sometimes in positions of significant authority. Finally, as institutions for the treatment and attempted cure of the mentally ill, asylums were designed to support domesticity and comfort, however vain their efforts in the face of budgets and overcrowding. This book will represent the material environment of the early nineteenth-century lunatic asylum and seek to address the historical reputation that the earliest asylums have gained, presenting them as pioneering rather than retrograde, even in the face of failure.

Acknowledgements

This book was made possible through the support of many people. Special thanks to Eleanor Casella, Julie-Marie Strange, Melanie Giles, Sian Jones, and Audrey Horning, without whose insight into my research and writing I could never have written this book. I am very grateful for the support of the Society for Post-Medieval Archaeology whose small research grant funded research in this book on the Lincoln Asylum. Vital feedback on the core research in this book was offered by several people in the British and Irish archaeological community at conferences and symposia, for which I am grateful. My research was facilitated by the staff, past and present, of several hospitals, particularly St Brendan's Hospital Dublin, St Fintan's Hospital Portlaoise, and the Stephen Beaumont Museum of Mental Health, to whom I owe much thanks. I also owe thanks to John Dunne for sharing photographs of the Maryborough Asylum with me.

I wish to thank the staff at the archive offices, local and national, who provided assistance while carrying out this research. I am very grateful to the people I worked with at Allen Archaeology in Lincoln for introducing me to the archaeology of the city, and to my former colleagues at the University of Sheffield for their encouragement and insight into my research when I worked there and after I left. For their valuable feedback, I am enormously obliged to my colleagues at the University of Lincoln, in particular Christine Grandy, Helen Smith, Adam Page, and Chris O'Rourke, for their historian's-eye view on my research.

I am extremely grateful to my friends for taking the time to talk to me about my work. I owe each and every one of you a drink. Particular thanks must go to Duncan Wright for his comments on the first drafts of this book. Thanks to Sarah Longair for hosting me in Venice while I was writing up some of this research, for many post-writing drinks, and for introducing me to Italian football. I owe thanks to Charlotte Newman, Deirdre Forde, and Suzanne Lilley for sharing their unique approaches to institutions and built heritage, which have informed my own approach.

Special thanks also to Thomas Sharp, Patrick Doyle, and the old Picnic Wednesdays crew. I made use of several good coffee shops and their wifi while preparing this manuscript, and owe particular thanks to the Angel Coffee House in Lincoln for excellent coffee, delicious cake, and a comfortable place to write.

    I am extremely grateful to my husband James Greenhalgh for his feedback on my research, his comments on drafts of my writing, for fostering a supportive and loving environment for me to do my work, and for his unfailing friendship. I was supported in writing this book by my family, whose faith and belief in me has been a keystone in my personal and professional life. Thanks to my sister Hannah, my brothers Shane and Michael, my sister-in-law Yvonne, my niece Mia, and my uncles Gerard, Micheal, and Kieran. Thanks also due to Tyler and Stacey for their companionship on many walkover surveys. My mother Kathleen Fennelly (neé Kelly) was my strongest supporter, and along with my father, Sean, made it possible for me to pursue academic research as a career. In addition to their love and support, my parents also lent me their expertise as mental health professionals, which inspired me to write this book.

Table of legislation

	Title	Date
UK: 39. Geo.3, c.38	Act of Union (Ireland)	1800
UK: 40. Geo.3, c.69	Union with Ireland Act	1800
UK: 48. Geo.3, c.96	Act for the Better Care and Maintenance of Lunatics, being Paupers or Criminals in England	1808
UK: 59. Geo.3, c.127	Irish Lunatic Asylums for the Poor Act	1817
UK: 9. Geo.4, c.40	County Asylums Act 'An Act to amend the Laws for the Erection and Regulation of County Lunatic Asylums. And More Effectually to Provide for the Care and Maintenance of Pauper and Criminal Lunatics in England'	1828
UK: 9. Geo.4, c.41	Madhouses Act 'An Act to regulate the Care and Treatment of Insane Persons in England'	1828
UK: 1 & 2. Geo.4, c.33	An Act to Amend an Act passed in the Eleventh Year of the Reign of His late Magesty King George the Fourth, Intituled [sic] *An Act for Appropriating the Richmond Lunatic Asylum in Dublin to the Purposes of a District Lunatic Asylum* (1831)	1831
UK: 8 & 9. Vict., c.100	Lunacy Act. Provision for the Commissioners of Lunacy	1845
UK: 8 & 9. Vict., c.126	County Asylums Act	1845
UK: 20 & 21. Vict., c.71	Lunacy (Scotland) Act	1857
UK: 7 & 8. Eliz.2, c.72	An Act to Repeal the Lunacy and Mental Treatment Acts 1890 to 1930, and the Mental Deficiency Acts 1913 to 1938, and to Make Fresh Provisions with Respect to the Treatment and Care of Mentally Disordered Persons and with Respect to their Property and Affairs, and for Purposes Connected with Matters Aforesaid	1959

UK: 1990, c.9	Planning (Listed Buildings and Conservation Areas) Act	1990
Ireland: Number 19 of 1945	Mental Treatment Act	1945
Ireland: Number 30 of 2000	Planning and Development Act	2000
Ireland: Number 25 of 2001	Mental Health Act	2001
Council of Europe Treaty Series no. 143	European Convention on the Protection of the Archaeological Heritage (Revised), also known as the Malta Convention	1992

1

Introduction

The words 'lunatic asylum' conjure up images of imposing grey facades hiding white-washed corridors echoing with the torment of unwilling denizens. The popular association of these buildings with austerity and grimness has a long history. When an asylum was constructed outside the Irish town of Enniscorthy in Co. Wexford in the mid-nineteenth century, the surprisingly ornate architectural features of the institution gave rise to a local story. The story holds that the red-brick Italianate asylum building overlooking the picturesque Slaney Valley was originally planned as a palace, to be built in India rather than Ireland. In some (presumably) English colonial planning office, however, the plans for the ornate, Eastern palace were mixed up with those of an Irish asylum, the real building intended for Enniscorthy (National Inventory of Architectural Heritage 2019). The asylum, the story goes, was supposed to look like other, more austere and institutional-looking, asylums nearby without the elaborate architectural detail of the asylum as it was built.

Irish provincial asylums built in the 1820s and 1830s all shared a common architect and were built to similar (if not identical) plans. They were constructed from local stone, granite or limestone blocks, symmetrical and unadorned but for a cupola over the main administration block. The windows of an Irish provincial asylum were small and square and certainly did not boast flourishes like the Romanesque arches and carved stops which graced the Enniscorthy institution. The story of mixed-up plans at a busy London colonial office is not unique to Enniscorthy (or even to asylums), but that such local folklore should endure into the twenty-first century attests to the pervasiveness of popular expectations of these buildings, particularly those constructed in the nineteenth century. This story about the Enniscorthy Asylum makes a regular appearance in local media, and even in the Irish National Inventory of Architectural Heritage. The story has come to form part of the building's history, even if its veracity is questionable at best. Given the shadow cast by the legacy of two centuries of frequently experimental management practices in the treatment of the insane, the vague fiction of a more salubrious architectural heritage seems preferable to the idea that the asylum was only ever just that – an institution for confinement, however ornate its facade.

What stories like this one fail to acknowledge is that the form of lunatic asylum buildings, and buildings for confinement in general, was constantly reassessed, re-planned, and changed throughout the nineteenth century, according to the effectiveness of experimental new treatment methods and management practices, not to mention the vagaries of public works budgets. By the mid-nineteenth century, when the Enniscorthy Asylum was constructed, the architecture of the ideal public lunatic asylum had been a source of much debate for over half a century. Therefore, in order to trace the widely-held public opinion of asylums as austere, institutional, and utilitarian, it is necessary to go back to the early part of the nineteenth century, when a standard for large, public lunatic asylums at provincial level was still just a talking point in parliamentary committees. This book will explore the material structure and development of asylum buildings, examining the dichotomy between the progressive reform rhetoric inherent in their widespread construction in the early nineteenth century, and the practicalities of maintaining a large public institution in the face of massive overcrowding and increasing urban populations. In this manner, the book will trace the origins of the popular ideas of asylums as overcrowded, austere, and clinical, and propose an alternative view of these institutions as a public necessity, overtaxed by demand and lack of funds; as a workplace for the hundreds of people in areas of little industry; and, as much as was possible, a home for patients, for general staff, and for the individuals who ran them, the inheritance of whom is an active and living community of former staff and patients. What emerged from the early years of architectural and material experimentation was an imperfect but widespread and ordered system of provincial asylums across the British Isles, the basis for which lay in the trialling, successes, and failures of a few pioneering institutions.

Archaeology is a discipline concerned with the material legacy of social life. Archaeologists record the ways in which routine and ritual are carried out, changed, and abandoned over time, tracking the movement of people through landscapes using the things they leave behind. Archaeologists are thus well-placed to inform on changes in a busy land- and task-scape like the historic lunatic asylum. Lunatic asylums are rich archaeological sites, encompassing both buildings and landscapes, and can inform on the social, political, and economic life of the period in which they were built. Changes to the arrangement and use of asylum buildings are marked and (usually) leave visible traces in the material, if not always the documentary, record. Indeed, where the historical sources might only record a short building programme, or an increased number of patients, the impact of those changes in the material record can be as dramatic as a new wing to the building, or the reduction of outdoor space for patient recreation. Changes in the building's arrangement could have a significant impact on the ways in which the building was used and usurp the intentions of the architects and planners in ways that are rarely recorded explicitly.

So, what does an archaeology of lunacy look like? While lunacy in the past was not exclusively institutional, the study of historic asylums allows for a quantitative survey of the ways in which lunacy was conceived of and treated. This study of the subject of lunacy and asylums focuses, therefore, on the archaeology of those institutions where lunacy was managed within a framework: the asylums. Approaches to this subject in the United States and Australia have drawn heavily on historical documentation, as well as excavation data (where possible) and standing building survey. If archaeology is 'concerned with the physical and material aspects of past lives', as Sarah Tarlow has asserted (2007: 29), the archaeology of lunacy is a material and physical exploration of the lives of the builders, theorisers, and inhabitants of the historic asylum. In addition to material culture, cartographic sources also inform on site how sites developed and the spatial relationship between different elements of the site, or the host population, allowing for a broader exploration of how the inhabitants and proprietors of asylums negotiated a relationship with the people and spaces outside the walls. An archaeology of lunacy is, by necessity, multidisciplinary, drawing on the large body of evidence. This includes archival evidence for asylum governance at local and national level, cartography and visual sources like photographs and drawings, and the sites themselves, analysis of which can draw on archaeological approaches to landscapes, buildings, and material culture. Employing a multidisciplinary approach, this book will explore the landscapes and building of lunatic asylums in England and Ireland in the early nineteenth century.

Public lunatic asylums were constructed in the first half of the nineteenth century in England and Ireland under the aegis of the British Government. Following a series of Acts and parliamentary enquiries, discussed in detail in this chapter, the British Government was concerned with the construction of asylums which would reflect increasingly popular ideas about the management of the insane. The history of madness and medicine does not exist in a vacuum; the construction of large-scale public institutions for the confinement of the insane coincided with the first sallies of the Industrial Revolution. In many ways, lunacy in its modern form was a particular problem of the industrial age. People who could not work and contribute meaningfully to the increasingly industrial economy did not fit into a model for ideal behaviour. Added to this, a surge in the urban population meant that traditional frameworks for managing the insane at familial or community level broke down, and lunacy became a problem for the state. For this reason, many asylums constructed in the first decades of the nineteenth century were experimental in design or bore striking resemblance to other institutions for public confinement. With limited reference points for how an asylum, let alone a reformed asylum, should look, architects and reformers experimented. The result was a mix of different architectural styles, combining popular and effective designs for prisons and workhouses with the arrangement or setting of veteran's hospitals, factories, and country houses, among other institutions or large buildings. The resultant institution, the Georgian lunatic asylum, in turn informed its successors, the massive Victorian and Edwardian lunatic asylums which form the bulk of this kind of architectural heritage. Despite their myriad problems, which will be explored in this book, the public asylums built in the first half of the nineteenth century came to define the form, the management practice, and the architectural style of buildings for the confinement of the insane.

The lunatic asylum in historical context

Purpose-built lunatic asylums were a primarily urban phenomenon, and reasonably rare at the turn of the nineteenth century. The care of the insane prior to the construction of large public institutions fell to families or communities or small church-run institutions. Those who could not be cared for at home were managed by organised relief work or left in the charge of workhouses and prisons (Porter 2004: 125–7). If an individual or their family could afford to pay the (frequently steep) rates, a lunatic could be entrusted to the care of enterprising mad doctors who operated privately run madhouses. Private doctors began constructing private institutions in country house estates on an increasing scale from the mid-eighteenth century, responding to calls from the upper and middle classes for a more formal approach to the care of lunatics, particularly those who did not fall into the pauper class. Awareness of the plight of the lunatic was likely brought about when it became public knowledge that the king, George III, was himself so afflicted. Bethlem Hospital in London was a rare and famous example of a purpose-built public lunatic asylum in the early modern period and was not suitable for large numbers of fee-paying patients of the noble class, let alone a king.

By no means the only dedicated lunatic asylum in the city of London, Bethlem was distinctive. It is distinguishable from other asylums built before 1800 for both its antiquity and its dedication to the lower classes. Bethlem was a public asylum serving the needs of the city of London, with medieval monastic origins and a historical reputation for the charitable reception of the insane – though better accommodation was also available for a fee. The hospital grew out of the Priory of St Mary Bethlehem which garnered a reputation in the later Middle Ages for taking in lunatics. The situation of the hospital, on the main highway leading north out of the city, meant that it was in an ideal position to solicit alms from passers-by (Andrews *et al*. 1997: 36). Though swiftly overtaken by the rapidly expanding city, Bethlem set an early precedent for the situation of future asylums: in removed – quieter – spaces outside, but close, to large population centres. As well as the insane, the hospital also took in the sick and the destitute, some of whom died while in the Priory. Excavations of the Priory burial ground undertaken by the Museum of London Archaeology on behalf of Crossrail in 2015 revealed over three thousand burials on the site, including a mass grave dating to a sixteenth- or early seventeenth-century plague outbreak (Crossrail 2017), likely in use when the Priory was still in operation. This shows that the site was a focal point for the destitute for all manner of ailments, and for the poor in times of crisis. It is not surprising, therefore, that the site became increasingly overcrowded.

When the Bethlem Hospital was relocated to a new site in Moorfields in 1676, it was rebuilt in a large, purpose-built institution, a 'palace beautiful' for the mad, far removed from the piecemeal architecture of the original Priory site (Arnold 2008: 87). The baroque architecture of the new Bethlem Hospital marked a shift in attitude towards the insane. Madness was no longer seen as a divine punishment or moral affliction, and the new hospital indicated a move towards the idea of a dedicated institutional framework to support the deserving mad – a purpose-built space that was visually and operationally separate from a prison or workhouse (Philo 2004: 432). Unfortunately, overcrowding soon marred the noble intentions of the Moorfields hospital. The word 'bedlam' – to mean uproar and confusion – comes from the popular rendering of the asylum name, Bedlam, and its introduction into common parlance goes some way towards communicating how the public felt about the hospital. To support growing demand and a rapidly expanding urban population, Bethlem was relocated again in 1815 to a site in St George's Fields, this time to a classical-style building with a prominent portico and dedicated wings to promote patient classification. Patient classification according to severity and type of illness, as well as gender and status (fee-paying or not), was part of a wider trend in asylum building in the British Isles, North America, and across the Empire; a refinement in thinking about madness which called for specialised care for the mad according to the specific needs of the patient. This change in outlook – an increased emphasis on reform and improvement – was not limited to lunatic asylums, but was reflected in social, economic, and political life in this period. Linked to the ideas of progress and secular principles of independence and order which emerged from seventeenth- and eighteenth-century European intellectual enlightenment, the reform of lunatic asylums must be seen as part of what historian Asa Briggs referred to as an 'Age of Improvement' (2000: 2). This period was characterised by an increasing intersection between the ideas of human progress and improvement, the landscape, wealth, and labour – epitomised in *The Wealth of Nations,* a foundational text on political economy by Scottish economist Adam Smith (1776; Tarlow 2007: 22). In his book, *Madness and Civilisation*, Michel Foucault goes further to situate the change in thinking about lunacy within a more general 'Great Confinement': the separation and institutionalisation of those who could not contribute to the new industrialising economy (2006: 43). The scale of the new state-sponsored institutions and their aesthetic gravitas and monumentality supports Foucault's interpretation of these institutions as mechanisms of state power. This change was marked in management practices as well as aesthetics. The new Bethlem Asylum represented a visual and material shift away from the eighteenth-century urban madhouse. Located on a plantation on a site still on the fringes of the city, the Bethlem Asylum was a new type of institution, where fresh air was as important to the management of the insane as security. The new type of asylum that emerged at the end of the eighteenth century, as articulated in the new Bethlem Asylum, was built after the ideals of moral management.

The construction of large-scale public lunatic asylums in the early nineteenth century occurred within a shifting geographical framework of urban and rural consolidation and change and social development. A surge in population in the United Kingdom and Ireland during the eighteenth century drove urban development and the expansion of towns, while agricultural innovations and changes in farming practices in the countryside altered rural landscapes. As stated above, asylums were part of a much larger drive towards social and spatial improvement in this period, marked in the landscape and streetscape. In addition to increasing overcrowding and consequent health concerns in cities, fashion also played a part in changing how cities looked in this period. Continental trends towards wide streets and open amenity spaces in cities influenced massive changes to urban streetscapes in the British Isles from the late eighteenth century. The proliferation of a spirit of civic improvement throughout the British Isles is clearly articulated in the adoption of 'improving' principles in the city of Dublin before and after joining the Union in 1801. While different social, political, and religious concerns meant that Ireland and the United Kingdom were different in many ways (Tarlow 2007: 28–9), in the aesthetics of monumental and state architecture they became increasingly similar. The late Georgian period saw the creation of open squares, architectural vistas, and promenade streets in both London and Dublin (Craig 1982: 243; Nord 1988: 165), as well as the construction of increasingly regular street patterns in new industrial cities like Manchester and Edinburgh. In the countryside, agricultural land was enclosed into ordered, manageable estates; fields were arranged in straight-edged land parcels bordered by fences and hedges which irrevocably altered movement through the landscape and consolidated and specialised agricultural practices. Unproductive borders and margins were 'waste', while productively farmed fields were likened to industry. In the language of improvement, as in the public institution – the asylum and the workhouse – the idle or wasteful were contrary to the productive and industrial (Porter 2001: 309). Though land was enclosed ostensibly for economic purposes, the status inherent in owning an improved estate marked landowners out as forward thinking (Williamson 2007: 6) and modern. Historian Asa Briggs terms this movement towards modernity as the 'Age of Improvement' (as stated above), arguing that the spirit of progress which began with the European Enlightenment inspired moral, economic, technological, civic, rural, and urban improvements (Briggs 2000: 2).

Alongside the spirit of social improvement was a broader cultural acceptance, from the early modern period, of the need for the 'confinement' of those elements of the population which were not conducive to maintaining the economic and urban peace or contributing meaningfully to the betterment of society. These elements included the unemployed, the poor, the criminal, and the insane (Foucault 2006: 43–50; Tarlow 2007: 136). Those who could not work and contribute meaningfully to the industrial economy were a problem to be solved, or at least managed (Foucault 2006: 43). In the case of the mad, this process of management involved the construction of more comprehensive and effective asylums, from around the middle of the eighteenth century, in which the mad could be confined. Building on the success or imperative of expanding eighteenth-century asylums, more were constructed. The early nineteenth century was a period of considerable social and political upheaval, necessitating the formalisation of a means of managing the non-industrious population. The Napoleonic Wars had a significant impact on the British economy – as both a driver of new markets and a barrier to others. This impact continued throughout the conflict, and even after. In addition to a couple of bad harvests, Napoleon's blockades of British trade routes led to a period of economic crisis in 1811 and 1812. Thousands of people claimed poor relief during this period (Briggs 2000: 165), and there was significant strain on those institutions dedicated to the relief of the poor: on poorhouses, almshouses, and workhouses. After the war, the labour market was flooded with young men who had previously found employment in the army or the navy. As the population of able-bodied poor grew, institutions were strained. It is no coincidence that in the years in which many provincial asylums were planned, between 1808 and 1820, other, less specialised, institutions suffered significant overcrowding. Asylums relieved the burden of caring for the lunatic poor, a significant portion of the workhouse population.

Institutional confinement on a large scale was realised in (albeit elaborate and occasionally stylish) monolithic architecture, the buildings themselves expressions of public order represented in the monumental architecture of the day. One of the more explicit examples of this building type was Richmond Penitentiary in Dublin, nicknamed the 'Cease to do Evil Hotel' by locals and inmates for the inscription over the frontage which read 'Cease to do Evil, Learn to do Well' (O'Donnell 1972: 152–3). Though less austere or outwardly punitive, asylums built in this period were also constructed in a monumental style. The early nineteenth-century asylums were usually neo-classical, similar in form and scale to the rural dwelling-places of the upper classes. This style was popular in the architecture of hospitals for physical ailments too, such as the Dublin Lying-in Hospital, built in 1745, whose portico-adorned facade was comparable with the contemporaneously constructed palatial urban residence of James Fitzgerald, twentieth Earl of Kildare (Boyd 2006: 43–6). This was not a nineteenth-century phenomenon, but rather a large-scale realisation of a theme in hospital and asylum architecture from the early modern period from which asylum architects drew their inspiration. The architecture of public health in the early modern period was at times so impressive that it was mistaken for domestic architecture; for example, in an eighteenth-century guide to London, the hospital for invalids in Chelsea was described by author Edward Hatton as having the appearance of a palace, rather than a home for pensioners (1708: 737).

The neo-classical style and country-house architecture of public institutions correlated well with the growth in popularity of reformed and 'moral' styles of management. Moral management was not a single management practice, but rather a collection of doctrines, ideals, and practices which advocated for the management of the insane in a humane and caretaking manner. Management of the mad was a solution to the problem of confinement without an end. Moral management of the insane was conceived of against an increasingly secular backdrop of reason and individuality, born out of the European intellectual Enlightenment (Porter 1995: 264; Williams 1999: 7), an increasing acknowledgement of the use of logic and reason to solve the problems of the world; the problem of long-term confinement addressed through the logical and reasonable methods of enlightened men. In prisons, the introduction of reform as the ultimate goal for prisoners, over punishment, is one such improving principle of enlightened institutional management. Architecturally, the creation of an environment which reflected the principles of sanity, reason, and domestic comfort could, logically, promote sane, rational, and civilised behaviour. As regards the management and treatment of the insane, the term 'moral management' referred to a variation on *traitment moral*, the introduction of intelligence and passion into the consideration of treatment for the insane as espoused by French asylum reformer Phillippe Pinel and defined by his student, Jean-Étienne Esquirol (Kelly 2008b: 20; Tucker 2007: 118). Moral management in practice was the treatment of the mind in a logical and calm manner, encouraging patients to develop self-control with the assistance and support of a doctor and a wider institutional framework (Yanni 2007: 24), with minimal use of physical restraint.

In the British Isles, the principles of moral management were championed by men like Samuel Tuke, the manager of a private asylum, the York Retreat. Tuke promoted moral management through the publication of instructional texts on the management and construction of an asylum based on his own experience and expertise. Tuke's book, *Description of the Retreat* (1813), was one of several didactic texts on asylum design and management in the nineteenth century. The earliest of these texts were descriptive in nature, offering examples of best practice rather than explicit guidance on how asylums should be run (as with later texts, such as W.A.F. Browne's *What Asylums Were, Are and Ought to Be* [1837] or John Conolly's *The Construction and Government of Lunatic Asylums and Hospitals for the Insane* [1847]) (Browne 1991; Conolly 1847; Piddock 2007: 29–30). Like Tuke, Lincoln Asylum's Edward Parker Charlesworth used his own asylum to promote the adoption of his system of non-restraint, that is the abolition of mechanical restraints like chains and manacles in favour of solitary confinement and other, less punitive measures. His book, *Remarks on the Treatment of the Insane*, like Tuke's book, included a detailed annotated plan of his own asylum (1828). The architecture of the asylum was as intrinsic to the treatment of the insane as any management method. In Ireland, moral management advocates like William Saunders Hallaran, physician to the Cork City Asylum, also penned observational texts; Hallaran's *Practical Observations on the Causes and Cure of Insanity* (1818) was a detailed description of the application of moral management methods. Hallaran's book contained drawings of some of the instruments employed in his asylum, including a circulating swing and a leather brace. These instruments were to be alternatives to the manacles and chains of asylums of the past, and evidence the highly experimental nature of this period in the management of the insane.

Beginning in the early nineteenth century, a number of reform-inspired purpose-built lunatic asylums were constructed in Britain and Ireland. These asylums were administered at county level, and the various management practices implemented therein were drawn from the principles and ideals of moral management as preached by men like Tuke. A legislative framework for lunacy supported the construction of these asylums. A series of acts in the first half of the nineteenth century legislated for the construction of public lunatic asylums in England and Wales, and later established a centralised system of governance of asylums under a Commission. These acts were the County Asylums Act of 1808 (48. Geo.3, c.96), the County Asylums Act and Madhouses Act of 1828 (9. Geo.4, c.40; 9. Geo.4, c.41, respectively), and the Lunacy Act of 1845 (8 & 9 Vict. c.126). The 1808 Act, the first, made provision for the establishment of asylums at county level. The necessity of an asylum in a county was judged by local magistrates (Bewley 2008: 6; Smith 1999: 23). The 1828 Act went further, making the establishment of an asylum in each county compulsory, so that those counties which did not construct an asylum under the 1808 Act were compelled to do so. The 1845 Acts then formalised and centralised the new system of provincial and urban asylums under a single administrating body, through the creation of the Commissioners of Lunacy.

Lunatic asylums in Ireland were legislated for under a different system, and the system of provincial asylums was administrated centrally from the outset. Prior to the construction of purpose-built provincial asylums in the 1820s and 1830s, the insane were housed in a variety of institutions. Lunatic wards were established in houses of industry (workhouses) under the authority of the Inspector General of Prisons (Kelly 2014: 56). Even so, specialised institutional provision for the insane was largely urban in nature. In rural areas, the insane were cared for at home, or ended up in prisons or local infirmaries. Private asylums were relatively rare. The two largest urban institutions for the insane, St Patrick's Hospital and the Richmond Lunatic Asylum, were located in Dublin, Ireland's largest city. St Patrick's Hospital was established in 1747, paid for with a bequest from the Irish author Jonathan Swift (Figure 1.1). It was not a large asylum, and its plan by architect George Semple was based on the seventeenth-century Bethlem Hospital site at Moorfields (Reuber 1996: 1180). The original building was not large

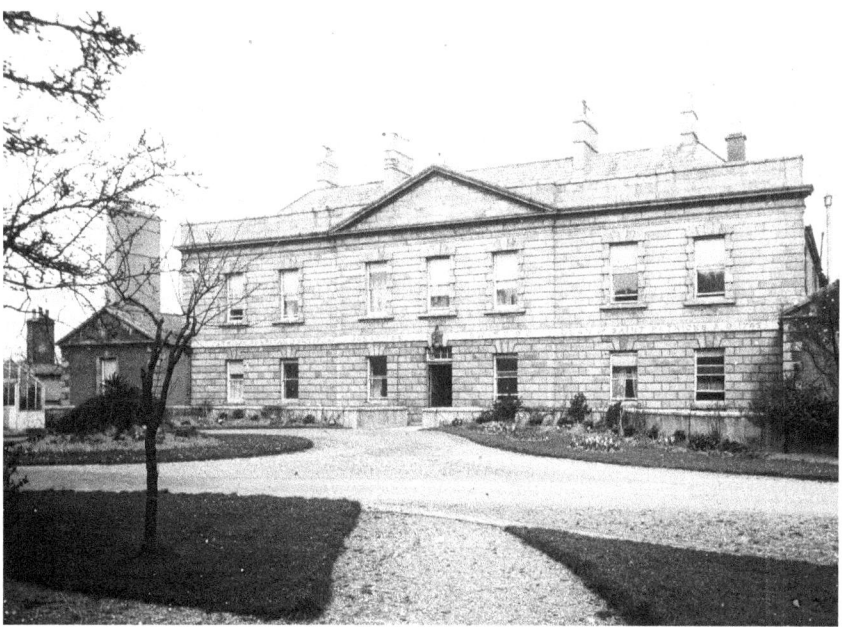

Figure 1.1 Facade of St Patrick's Hospital, Dublin (c. 1890–1910).

enough to meet demand and further accommodation for the insane was added over the course of the eighteenth century. Francis Johnston, who would later design the Richmond Asylum and subsequent provincial asylums, worked as assistant to the architect Thomas Cooley on additions to the hospital in 1778. His experience with this asylum heavily informed his later institutional works. As such, St Patrick's early modern architecture had a significant influence on the form which the early nineteenth-century asylums took. The Richmond Lunatic Asylum was built as an addition to the Dublin House of Industry and opened in 1817. Overcrowding in both asylums indicated that provision for the insane was not sufficient in two large urban asylums, even with the support of various provincial houses of industry and prisons. The Irish Lunatic Asylums for the Poor Act of 1817 (59. Geo.3, c.127) supported the establishment of a dedicated district asylum to be constructed in each of Ireland's four provinces: Leinster (outside the city of Dublin), Munster, Connacht, and Ulster. By the 1820s, a more comprehensive system was devised to reflect the demographics of provincial Ireland, and nine provincial asylums were eventually built. The implementation of this organised system was overseen by a Board of General Control and, unlike the county-based system in England, was administered centrally from Dublin.

As asylums in England and Ireland were constructed regularly and disparately from 1808, and without a centralised administration (until 1817 in Ireland, and 1845 in England), instructive publications on the design and correct management of a reformed moral asylum were widespread, penned primarily by physicians but also by architects and asylum managers. Different architectural styles were matched with management practices, each with their own variations and interpretations of moral management and non-restraint. The individual personalities and preferences of asylum managers and visiting physicians were reflected in how asylums were run. This early period of public asylum building, from the County Asylums Act in 1808 to the Lunacy Acts in 1845, was a period of significant experimentation.

The mid-1840s marked a shift in the administrative structure of asylums in the British Isles, with the establishment of the Commissioners of Lunacy to replace the local magistrates in English and Welsh asylums and the Board of General Control in Ireland. The 1845 Lunacy Acts initiated a surge of asylum building, which required regulated, centralised administration and a relative degree of uniformity in design. The ideas for these designs, however, were drawn from asylums constructed before 1845, during those years of experimentation in architecture and management. As such, these asylums occupy a place of significant influence in the built history of lunatic asylums. Despite the influence which these buildings had, however, much of the secondary literature on asylum construction has been focused on asylums built after 1845 (see, for examples: Rutherford 2005, 2008; Stevenson 2000; Taylor 1995; Thompson and Goldin 1975; Yanni 2007). Among others, the West Riding Asylum at Wakefield, the Richmond Asylum in Dublin, and the Middlesex County Asylum were strong architectural models on which the regulated system was built. Middlesex was particularly influential, as the asylum management reformer and didactic author John Conolly was based there when he penned his popular treatise on the ideal asylum building: *The Construction and Government of Lunatic Asylums and Hospitals for the Insane* (1847). The asylums constructed after the 1845 Acts, in the wake of Conolly's treatise and very much informed by it – the large Victorian lunatic asylums – have come to dominate the history of asylum architecture. Innocuous in the English and Irish landscape, these massive buildings have become the archetypical asylum building, eclipsing the institutions which came before.

By the end of the twentieth century, many of the large asylums – those constructed in the first wave of asylum building before 1845 and those constructed after – ceased operation as hospitals or facilities for the poor. Many were closed, others repurposed, and a few were demolished or left exposed to weather and vandalism. The result of this mass closure was that dozens of large institutional buildings in English and Irish towns and cities stood empty and in need of reuse. Given the architectural merits of the buildings, many have been listed, preventing complete demolition. The buildings that remain present an ideal opportunity to study the architecture of the early management of the insane. Not all have been abandoned, however; some asylum buildings have been redeveloped, presenting interesting archaeological case studies in themselves. The ways in which asylum buildings have been redeveloped are telling of the stigma attached to mental health and twenty-first-century ideas about nineteenth-century madness. Repurposing has not been without its concerns, from a heritage perspective. These buildings pose significant challenges for developers, including the extent of the listing, the condition of the building and materials, the accessibility of the building from nearby locales, and the historic reputation of former asylums. The mitigation of this latter concern is clearly evidenced by the renaming of the buildings, redevelopment of the landscape and approaches, and in a few rare cases the use of the redeveloped buildings for the purposes of entertainment. This has included the use of former asylum buildings as filming locations or as 'haunted' attractions. The 'dark' heritage – associated with human suffering or death – of former lunatic asylum buildings and their frequent grouping with prisons and workhouses has impacted their study as built heritage, as well as their development. Indeed, the problematic legacy of the buildings has overshadowed their role as large-scale employers, suppliers, customers, venues for community building, and dwelling places, with the result that redevelopment rarely considers the impact of a modified landscape or rebranding on the historic communities which have grown up around these buildings.

Approaches to the historic asylum

In this book, the historic lunatic asylum will be approached as an archaeological, material landscape. Asylums extended beyond the physical boundaries of the buildings proper and were embedded into the semi-rural plantations in which they were situated, as well as the wider, increasingly urbanising landscapes of Britain and Ireland. A non-traditional approach to archaeology is required for the study of these sites, as formal excavation and material-culture study in situ is not always possible where buildings are still standing, sites are closed, or former asylum buildings have been put to alternative use (Newman 2016). The approach to the archaeological landscape and built heritage of the lunatic asylum outlined in this book builds on an existing base of scholarship on the archaeology of lunacy and lunatic asylums, as well as archaeological approaches to other institutions for confinement. The historic lunatic asylum was part of a wider drive towards social improvement, which included the construction of many forms of institution for social control. As such, this study draws on archaeological approaches to other institutions constructed during this period. Rooting this study in the archaeology of historical institutions allows for cross comparison with other contemporaneous institutions, showing the wider context for the innovations and motivations of asylum builders and managers.

There have been several notable studies on the archaeology and built heritage of historic asylums which I have drawn on in this book. Susan Piddock's book on lunatic asylums in Australia and Britain firmly roots 'institutional archaeology' as an emerging field in historical archaeology, deriving from socially-focused feminist approaches to archaeology and material culture (2007: 8). Seeking to contribute to this emerging field of institutional archaeology, this study draws on Piddock's effective application of archaeological principles, methods, and theory to the study of asylum buildings, in which she establishes a clear method for the critical and comparative use of documentary evidence and historic built heritage. Given the breadth of published literature from the early nineteenth century on how asylums *should* look, it is necessary when studying these buildings to evaluate the material as well as documentary evidence in order to ascertain how the complex ideas of asylum builders and reformers were actually put into practice. Piddock demonstrates how the comparative use of documentary and material sources can ascertain the challenges posed by individual sites, building materials, or the constraints of local authorities in implementing written ideas on the ground (2007). Piddock's book has a broad remit, focusing primarily on those asylums constructed in the second half of the nineteenth century. This study therefore builds on Piddock's examination by taking in asylums constructed in the first wave of large-scale asylum building and exploring Irish, as well as British, examples.

In this book, the archaeology of lunacy will be addressed in the context of a public institution: the district lunatic asylum. The archaeology of lunacy in the nineteenth century is not confined to the public asylum, however, and this study will also draw on non-institutional archaeologies. Sunshine Psota's materially focused examination of mental illness in domestic assemblages, for example, explored the ways in which insanity can be identified through material culture, including medicine bottles (2011). In this book I will use similar types of material culture, notably cutlery and ceramics, to explore how individual asylums imposed authority on patients and staff alike. As with this study, Psota's approach was interdisciplinary, comparing the domestic material with the casual admission records of mental health institutions. Though public asylums housed patients on a long- and short-term basis, long-term patients were frequently the focus of contemporaneous didactic texts on asylums in the early nineteenth century and remain a central focus in histories of medicine. This is perhaps due to the point that casual or short-term patients were less likely to succumb to the mindset of institutionalisation, a social integration into the asylum due to habit and context while in long-term residence that makes leaving the institution a source of anxiety and fear, as theorised by anti-psychiatry sociologist Erving Goffman (1976: 69). Short-term patients are thus harder to identify in the material record. Short-term patients comprised a larger portion of the patient population in private asylums than in public asylums. As such, this study does take account of archaeological studies of lunacy in private institutions for comparative purposes. Private asylums were impacted as much by reformed ideas on the treatment and management of the insane as public asylums. In her examination of the private asylum Brooke House in Chiswick, London, Charlotte Newman (2015) identified decorative practice and interior arrangement as facets of treatment. Newman made effective use of a curated collection of interior decoration held by English Heritage, and in her comparative approach to both material culture and the documentary record demonstrated the potential of both to offer a broad view of how spaces for the treatment of lunacy developed over time. These archaeological studies on the material culture, architecture, and practical management of madness evidence the potential for a materially focused approach to inform on the daily life of an individual or an institution which is otherwise only represented in the official historical record.

Asylums in the British Isles, which are the focus of this study, are representative samples of how institutions could develop in an industrialising landscape. Despite their similarities, however, each individual asylum was constructed according to the constraints, limitations, and opportunities of the geographic and social contexts in which they were built. This book draws on approaches taken in archaeological studies of asylums in colonial contexts to draw out regionality, such as Peta Longhurst's critical comparison of ideology and the built environment in New South Wales, Australia (2015). Longhurst drew on existing scholarship on the archaeology of institutions to effectively apply theories of non-correspondence (the idea that the interplay between social action and the material world is not deterministic, as theorised by archaeologist Roland Fletcher) to asylums in New South Wales, populating the historic asylum with social actors who actively engaged with their environment. Identifying the ways in which individuals approached their material world is essential in an archaeological approach to institutions, as the relative homogeneity of architectural plans and a plethora of didactic texts on ideal asylum environments can suggest commonality where there is significant material difference.

Lunatic asylums were not constructed in isolation, but as part of a wider drive of institutional reform and welfare, as previously discussed. Asylum buildings share much in common with prisons and workhouses, which were frequently constructed under the same governing bodies or by the same architect. While asylums had a different mission and remit than prisons or workhouses, they share many similar features in terms of management, in particular an attention towards the reform and self-governance of the inmate. In light of these commonalities, this study will draw heavily on other institutional archaeologies. From their construction, reformed public asylums in the nineteenth century practised the classification of patients, and space within the asylum was ordered according to patient diagnoses, gender, and class. This careful organisation of space according to use was one aspect of British social and domestic life which made its way into institutions. In her work on Magdalene asylums – institutions for the reform of 'fallen women' – in Philadelphia, archaeologist Lu Ann De Cunzo identified this spatial organisation as an aspect of 'moral' life outside the institution which was co-opted into its architecture (2001: 27). The moral life of the patient was key to the type of management that reformers like the York Retreat's Samuel Tuke were aspiring to, and the influence of domestic space on asylum architecture and management will be addressed in this book.

The theme of classification and segregation into dedicated spaces runs throughout the primary source material for asylums. The plans and descriptions of asylums by their financiers and architects are useful tools in identifying how the buildings were intended to function. Archaeology, as a discipline concerned with uncovering the material traces of human behaviour, offers an approach to the material remains that allows for the identification of resistance in these spaces, too. Resistance, on the part of the staff or the inmate to the intentions of the asylum authorities and their rules, is the action of an individual. As such, the material and historical traces of resistance, where they can be found, indicate human agency. The assertions of Michel Foucault regarding resistance, power, and domination in an institutional context (1991; 2006), and the impact of institutionalisation articulated by sociologist Erving Goffman (1976), have been applied in this study and guide critical analysis of the historical record. The ideas of Foucault, and to a lesser extent of Goffman, have been influential in the history and archaeology of madness, informing interpretations of the architecture and management of lunatic asylums from the late eighteenth century to the twentieth century. In his 1961 book, *Folie et déraison: Histoire de la folie à l'âge classique* – published in 1964 in English translation as *Madness and Civilisation*, as discussed above – Foucault asserted that the institutional confinement of the mad in the nineteenth century was a feature of industrialisation. Those who could not meaningfully engage with the 'imperative of labour' were necessarily confined in out-of-the-way places – asylums (2006: 43). Throughout his interpretation of asylums as repositories for inconvenient and unproductive people, he criticised men like Samuel Tuke and Philippe Pinel of Paris, both didactic authors on the subject of asylums. Foucault's criticising approach to their writing and the mission of asylum reformers informs critical reading in this study. However, Foucault's approach is itself flawed in that his reading of nineteenth-century institutions was coloured by his own intellectual context. Foucault, like Erving Goffman, was a key figure in the anti-psychiatry movement, an intellectual movement involving social commentators and academics, as well as psychiatrists and doctors, which challenged the use of physical methods and involuntary treatment, as well as the institutional confinement of the mentally ill, in the second half of the twentieth century. Goffman's primary focus was mental hospitals in the mid-twentieth century, but his ideas about institutionalisation have been influential in the history of medicine, and historians of medicine like Roy Porter have engaged with his work critically. As such, his work will be taken into account in this study, particularly with regards to the idea of the 'total institution'.

In his 1961 work, *Asylums*, Goffman posited that the key principle in the operation of a total institution, that is an institution catering to all aspects of an inmate's life (in this case, the mid-twentieth century mental hospital), is the institutionalisation of the inmate. In acculturation to the inner workings of an institutional life, an inmate becomes dependent on that culture and consequently suffers when faced with leaving it for the outside world (1976: 70–3). Porter has queried the application of Goffman's ideas to the Georgian lunatic asylum, suggesting that the units in question were, in that period, too small to be considered effective as total institutions (2004: 162). While agreeing with Porter that Goffman's principles of the total institution are too general to be applied wholesale to a system as inconsistent and small scale as the Georgian lunatic asylums, Goffman's assessment of the patient and staff experience of institutionalisation as key to the maintenance of order stands up to scrutiny. In this book, I will engage with this idea as it relates to discipline and resistance (see Chapter 3). This book seeks to challenge one common aspect of Foucault's interpretation and Goffman's critique: that the material environment of historic asylums is primarily punitive. In this study, I will argue that the interior layout of some of the earliest asylums evidences a caretaking attitude towards lunacy that can be seen in the architecture and material arrangement of asylums. This is not to suggest that resistance was not also a facet of everyday life in the asylum. For this reason, archaeological approaches to the theme of resistance in other institutions will be drawn on for comparative purposes.

The theme of resistance runs through several historical archaeologies of institutions for confinement, providing a rich body of research on which this study can draw. Eleanor Casella's work on prisons and penal colonies, in particular, demonstrates the potential of excavated material in showing that inmates operate beyond their proscribed roles. Casella's work on the Ross Female Factory in Tasmania, Australia accounts for the materiality of resistance uncovered through archaeological excavation. Excavated contraband artefacts, such as alcohol bottle glass and clay tobacco pipes in patient cells and in the prison grounds, suggest that clandestine behaviour and resistance to established hierarchies was common (2002, 2007). This approach to domination and resistance as articulated in the archaeological record has been applied in other institutional contexts such as internment and prisoner of war camps (Mytum and Carr 2013) and can be applied to lunatic asylums in excavated material and in the study of the built environment. Through excavated material and spatial analysis of built remains, the actions and behaviour of prisoners on a daily basis, largely absent from the official records of these institutions, is made visible. Spatial analysis and built heritage study will form the core methods of this book, rather than excavation. Despite this, resistance will still be addressed through the material remains.

Most nineteenth-century lunatic asylums in the British Isles are still standing in some form, and access to the sites is limited, if possible at all. A non-destructive means of studying the buildings and sites necessarily excludes any form of excavation. Archival sources such as cartography and building plans form a rich vein for studying these buildings archaeologically (as per Piddock 2007), while standing building survey techniques such as photographic survey and built-fabric analysis have been used to good effect in other institutional settings, such as Charlotte Newman's study of the Madeley Union Workhouse which explored the ways in which the institution of the mid-nineteenth-century workhouse responded to increasing industrialisation in a rural landscape (2013). However, standing building surveys on institutional sites are sometimes hampered by changes to the building fabric as a result of development. Lunatic asylum sites in the British Isles have been transformed into apartment buildings, markets, university buildings, and hotels. In consequence, original plasterwork is moved, and sometimes whole sections of the buildings are demolished, while sites are re-landscaped according to the needs of the new development. This kind of development is destructive to the original sites but also offers new opportunities for study not normally open to researchers. Archaeological site reports generated during development are key resources in these cases. Development-led archaeology on sites can answer questions about the past uses of the site. For example, excavations at the Lincoln Lunatic Asylum site after the closure of hospital in the 1980s uncovered the remains of a late-medieval church and high-medieval hospital on the site (Vince 2003: 307), indicating that the area where the asylum was constructed had a long history of institutional infrastructure. Records from these archaeological events, like site reports and desk-based assessments, are useful in assessing the long-term histories of individual sites. These records are easily accessible, if underused in academic research on these sites. Since 1990, archaeological remains are protected by law in the United Kingdom (Planning Act 1990, c.9). This covers scheduled monuments and listed buildings, and thus includes lunatic asylums. Developers and planners are bound to evaluate sites before development and adhere to guidance on the preservation of archaeological landscapes. Resulting reports from surveys of lunatic asylum sites are valuable resources in institutional archaeology. As a signatory to the 1992 European Convention on the Protection of the Archaeological Heritage (known as the Malta Convention or the Valetta Treaty) (Council of Europe Treaty Series no. 143), archaeological heritage is also a central planning concern in Ireland, where it is reinforced by national legislation (Number 30 of 2000). Large development-led excavations, like those undertaken at the Kilkenny Union Workhouse site in Ireland in 2006, offer valuable data on life in institutions. The 2006 excavation unearthed a graveyard associated with the workhouse which allowed for examination of diet and disease in the institution and offered valuable insights into privations at the workhouse during the Irish Famine of 1845–49 (Geber 2015). Peripheral aspects of institutional life, such as burial grounds, represent aspects of institutional life which are not always clear in the historical record. Grey literature – reports resulting from development-led archaeology on these sites – are invaluable resources for studying the long histories and changes on institutional sites.

Much scholarship on the spatial and material world of the historic lunatic asylum has been focused on the architecture of the buildings themselves, though the deliberate situation of these buildings in carefully chosen, curated parks and managed landscapes must be borne in mind when analysing them. Descriptive accounts of the buildings inform on how the architecture of mental health developed over time. These accounts, such as Jeremy Taylor's detailed overview of hospital architecture, asylum gardens, and landscaping (1991), are useful in creating a typology of the buildings and are used in this study to situate individual asylums within their wider stylistic context. More in-depth approaches to how the spaces were managed and the buildings functioned as lived places have been published since the early 1990s, and these more detailed spatial studies will be drawn from here. Asylum buildings were dynamic spaces, in which individual agents acted and reacted according to the ideology inherent in the institutions. Thomas Markus's studies of the spatial syntax of asylum spaces – that is the network of access routes, hierarchies of movement, and the use of space in the buildings (1993) – form a basis for the analysis of access and movement in this book. Markus's work is part of the body of asylum scholarship influenced by Foucault's ideas of power and confinement in the asylum (outlined above). This scholarship includes the edited volume on the built environment of mental healthcare, *Madness, Architecture, and the Built Environment* (Topp *et al.* 2007), which showcases approaches to lunatic asylums and mental health from geographical, social, and spatial perspectives. One aspect of asylum architecture which is featured in this collection, and numbers among the concerns of Markus in his work, is the idea of the panoptic gaze. This is the architecture of surveillance, and specifically of unseen, all-seeing vigilance on the part of the management of the asylum. The architectural panopticon, as proposed by Jeremy Bentham (1791), is referred to widely as a primary influence in the planning and design of asylums (see also, Franklin 2002b; Kennihan 2003; Markus 1993; Reuber 1996; and Richardson 1998). While Bentham's influence on the architecture of public institutions is undoubted given the frequency with which panoptic-style designs are referred to in didactic texts, government legislation, and articulated in asylum buildings themselves, the extent to which this design was put into practice is in question and will be addressed in this book.

The active management and movement of people through the lunatic asylum forms a core tenet of this study. As such, the interior make-up and furniture of the building will be addressed as inhibitive or reinforcing features of the lived asylum. This materially focused study builds on recent material approaches to the lunatic asylum, which have moved beyond the shell of the buildings and into the rooms themselves. Rather than cold or clinical spaces, nineteenth-century asylums were designed with ideas of domesticity and comfort in mind, and each asylum addressed this concern in its own way. Recent studies of institutional interiors from a historical perspective are drawn on here to explore this facet of asylum study. Jane Hamlett's work on institutional interiors moves away from presentations of institutions for confinement as homogenous or impersonal, and accounts for the adoption and use of domestic furnishings (2015). In her collaboration with Lesley Hoskins, they take this idea further to focus specifically on the aesthetic interior, on decoration in the public and private asylums as a feature of management and care in the later nineteenth century (2012). Similarly, in an archaeological approach to the therapeutic aesthetic of the private asylum, Charlotte Newman has posited that the use of unusual and expensive wallpapers contributed to the domestic environment (Newman 2016). These studies show the potential of a materially focused study in informing on how asylums were dynamically managed. Rather than timeless or static, asylums changed rapidly both inside and outside, according not only to pressures from overcrowding or wider changes in management practice, but also to fashion, taste, and social concerns. Focusing primarily on the early part of the nineteenth century, this book will bear both the local and wider context of asylums in mind when addressing the ways in which they changed over time. In terms of how these buildings developed over the two hundred years between their construction and their closure, the earliest phases of interior decoration are the least likely to survive into the present day.

Where original early nineteenth-century lunatic asylum buildings have survived into the present day, they are frequently part of larger hospital complexes, municipal buildings, commercial or residential buildings, or hotels. In consequence, while the buildings themselves survive, they are much altered and their wider landscape context is frequently changed beyond recognition. Despite the mass closure and repurposing of asylum buildings in Britain and Ireland in the second half of the twentieth century (see the Mental Health Acts (UK) 7 & 8. Eliz.2, c.72, and the 2001 Mental Health Act in Ireland, alongside a series of reports and proposals for change), a large number remain unoccupied or in a state of transition. How the buildings have been adapted for reuse has been contingent upon the inheriting body. From an archaeological perspective, redevelopment has had a significant impact on the heritage management of the material remains and reflects the social legacy of the institutions in general. Asylum buildings are divisive sites. On the one hand, major historic employers and institutions for community welfare within locales. On the other hand, asylums are frequently seen as sites of social control and hardship, where the worst of state and institutional neglect and privation was played out throughout the nineteenth and twentieth centuries. This reputation is not undeserved in many cases, though it is by no means universal. Alongside historic prisons and closed workhouses, asylum sites can be considered as sites of dark or difficult heritage. Asylums, as closed-door sites of mystery, have become a kind of cultural short-hand for suffering, and are frequently used in video games, in film, and in television as venues for horror and fear. Enduring public discomfort with mental illness into the modern period has, in many ways, been transferred to the material sites in which mental illness was treated. In their study of the phenomenon of dark tourism, John Lennon and Malcolm Foley cite film and television media as vehicles for popularising scenes of dark or difficult history, such as the sinking of the RMS *Titanic* and its portrayal in cinema throughout the twentieth century (2000: 17–18). Asylums are a particularly frequent reference point in fiction. The Danvers State Hospital, an 1870s state asylum in Massachusetts, for example, was an inspiration for horror writer H.P. Lovecraft's Arkham Sanitarium, the scene of a grisly patient murder in his short story, *The Thing on the Doorstep* (2018). In all of his writing, Lovecraft uses the buildings and landscapes of New England to create atmosphere (Evans 2004: 189). Lovecraft mentioned Danvers itself in his works, for example as the suspected final destination for ill-fated visitors to mysterious towns (see *The Shadow Over Innsmouth*; Lovecraft 2011: 274). Even in retirement (Danvers no longer operates as an asylum and has been partially demolished), this asylum has been unable to shake its reputation; in his essays on haunted buildings in the United States, Harry Skrdla references Danvers's influence on Lovecraft in the same context as he refers to the earlier history of the site as part of early modern Salem of witch-trial infamy (2006). These kinds of associations have a direct influence on how the built heritage of historic asylum buildings is treated once they cease operating as hospitals.

The cultural reference point of asylums as venues of horror both draws on and reinforces public discomfort with the built heritage of the historic lunatic asylum. Indeed, some have even become tourist attractions in themselves. As such, the dark legacy of both the sadly real and fantastically fictional needs to be considered when looking at the future of asylum buildings as built heritage, and even when arranging fieldwork for archaeological assessment of the sites. Laura McAtackney's work on the Maze/Long Kesh Prison in Northern Ireland (2014) is a good example of how archaeologists can approach buildings with difficult and conflicting histories. Her book is an archaeologically focused examination of the issues surrounding a problematic and politically volatile site of dark heritage. Her work is a model from which to study the dark and difficult legacy of institutions from an archaeological perspective. This book will contribute to the established, multidisciplinary literature on dark heritage and dark tourism, exploring the built environment of the nineteenth-century asylum throughout and offering a holistic approach to the material world of the historic lunatic asylum in its earliest period of large-scale development – the first half of the nineteenth century. The built heritage of the buildings will be revisited in the conclusion, with a short discussion on how a broader view of asylums, beyond the buildings themselves, may inform repurposing and preservation of this building type. In this way, this book will problematise the selective and inconsistent preservation of asylum buildings and difficult institutional built heritage in England and Ireland.

Methodology

The largely still-standing remains of the early nineteenth-century lunatic asylum system represent a unique opportunity, from an archaeological perspective, to study a building in active transition – materially and ideologically. It also makes their study, from an archaeological perspective, problematic. The conversion of asylum sites into apartment buildings, hotels, universities, and office blocks means that the grounds have already undergone intensive redevelopment in many cases. Commercial archaeology is a valuable source of excavation data on these sites, but the focus of commercial watching briefs, standing building surveys, and evaluations varies from site to site, dictated by the level of disruption to the built heritage. Where buildings have continued in use as psychiatric facilities, the privacy of patients limits what on-site work can be done (Piddock 2007: 29). As such, building survey was not always possible. This book employs methods drawn from archaeological landscape analysis, material culture study, and historical research.

The historic lunatic asylum was comprised of more than just a building for accommodation or a set of structures. Established on landscaped estates, often surrounded by planned gardens and plantations, the asylum was a complex made up, variously, of accommodation blocks, administration buildings, gate lodges, out-buildings, and utilities such as a laundry, a bake house, and a kitchen – and sometimes a farm. The asylum was both a landscape in the material sense that it was a complex physical space through which people move and relationships were established, and a taskscape in that each space was dedicated to an activity or interaction (as per Ingold 1993: 158). The successful operation of the asylum was dependent upon the maintenance of a social and spatial hierarchy, defined not just by the position of the individual – patient, keeper, doctor – but also their material signifiers; keepers, for example, carried keys. The social and spatial hierarchy of the asylum was also defined by privilege of movement and access. The maps and plans of historic lunatic asylums form the core primary and material source in this archaeology of lunacy, as they are informative of both the approved plan and original form of the historic asylum, as well as its redevelopment over time and the intention behind spatial division (if not always an accurate reflection of how people moved through the space in practice). Lines of sight, access points, and pathways for movement and sight were central to the management and operation of the asylum and were recreated using historical records and built heritage study. Asylum plans and maps of the local areas were cross-referenced with other sources, such as historic photographs and twentieth-century plans, as well as historical accounts and, where possible, standing building survey.

In order to study access and egress from the asylums as a stage in power relationships, relational graphs showing lines of movement and points of access were compiled for selected asylums. These graphs are a modified and simplified version of the spatial relationship graphs called *gamma maps*. Bill Hillier and Julienne Hanson theorised gamma maps and relational graphs in their 1984 book, *The Social Logic of Space*, as an articulation of three related principles present in almost all cases of spatial designs. These are that space should be hierarchically arranged, with a well-marked series of public-to-private zones. That the object of spatial layout is a physical expression of single-group identity and the exclusion of others; and that separate identity group spaces should be segregated from each other (Hillier and Hanson 1984: 130). The object of a gamma map is to demonstrate the control of space and access through the mapping of alpha (single entrance) and gamma (multiple entrances) spaces on a relational graph. While Hillier and Hanson's work can be criticised for being formulaic and presumptive of adherence to a social norm (and therefore discounting individual agency), their second summation – that spatial design in architecture demonstrates an articulation of identity and exclusion – can be used to discern intention in the design of buildings, if not in day-to-day practice. This method has been employed with success by Markus in his consideration of asylum architecture, in order to determine access and power in nineteenth-century institutions, specifically asylums in Scotland (1993). This book draws heavily on Markus's work. Markus's gamma maps illustrated the interior spatial structure and divisions within an institution, and demonstrated access and in some cases visual links, as in his spatial plan of the Edinburgh Bridewell (1989: 95). Markus's use of the maps to demonstrate visual links mirrors the work of James Delle (1998) and Terrance Epperson (2000), who used intervisibility, viewpoints, and viewsheds to illustrate panopticism, hierarchy, and power in archaeological landscapes. Intervisibility, viewpoints, and viewsheds, as well as movement, access, and spatial hierarchies were intrinsic to the success of moral management, as will be outlined in this book.

Spatial division and complex classification were essential features of the moral asylums, as will be outlined. The careful control of space was key to the maintenance of classifications and security. Historic asylums have frequently been seen as marginal spaces, not least by politician Enoch Powell in his speech to justify mass mental hospital closure in Britain in 1961. This idea of asylums as marginal, transitional, and in some cases 'sacred' or rarefied spaces will be revisited in this book. In his 1901 book, *Le rites de passage*, published in English as *The Rites of Passage* (1960), French ethnographer Arnold Van Gennep explored the practice of religion and social ritual through the organisation of space, specifically the spatial transition between profane and sacred, that is liminal space (1960). In this book, the lunatic asylum will be examined as a dedicated and protected (sacred) space, for which admission involved a complex series of bureaucratic and cleansing rituals. The dichotomy between 'profane' and 'sacred' may be identified in the classification and designation of internal and external, private and public space within the asylum. The hierarchy that dictated the privilege of access and movement through the site was supported by the maintenance of liminal spaces and stages: the admission office, the gate lodge, the front garden, and the visitors' rooms, to name a few. In this book, those liminal spaces will be explored, referred to as threshold spaces through which an actor must qualify to move. This means of reading spaces and spatial sources draws heavily on Van Gennep's concept of the threshold as a magico-religious space – a liminal space over which one must cross to alter identity. These ideas about liminality and identity will be applied to asylum architecture, historic plans and maps, and compared with historical sources for administration practice. The aim of this means of analysis is to identify the expectations and material environments necessary to carry out the rituals of everyday practice, namely movement, surveillance, admission, and discharge. Far from linear, these practices were heavily dependent on the creation and maintenance of a dedicated asylum environment and hierarchy.

Architectural histories of asylums have, in the past, focused on the visual and aesthetic features of the lunatic asylum. The carefully planned built environment on which both the success and failure of moral management depended, however, was more than just visual and decorative. This book will examine the physical environment of the asylum from a visual, sonic, and environmental perspective. Australian historian of medicine, Dolly MacKinnon, has suggested that the study of madness has been silent; the aural or sonic is overtaken in histories of the subject by the visual (Hilmes 2005: 249; MacKinnon 2003: 73). Study of the careful use and control of sound and acoustics as an aspect of place-making in the asylum contributes to the understanding of supervision and control of movement and space. Noise and its management in the nineteenth century have been considered an important feature of living in an increasingly urban environment. In his essay 'On noise', Hillel Schwartz illustrated the primary position of concern that background noise held in the nineteenth-century urban mindset, enough to see the introduction of Quiet Zones (2004: 51–3). Sonic features of the urban environment such as the church bell were key to the creation of industrialised mindsets and personal geographies; the church bell was both a timekeeper and a symbol of territorial identity (Corbin 2004: 184). Mackinnon pointed out that staff in historic asylums used bells and whistles in the early twentieth century in Australia in order to create a sense of time and regulation (2003: 76). The prominence of the whistle and the bell in museum collections for madness support the central role of these objects in the daily life of the asylum. However, it is difficult to assess the acoustic experience of the interior of an historical asylum. Mackinnon has utilised case notes and asylum histories in order to build an understanding of the interior soundscapes of these buildings. This book draws on these historical approaches to sound and contributes to the methodological framework for this study by examining unintentional noise, such as unlocking doors, footfalls, and rustling, as contributors to the creation of an institutional sonic environment.

There is an established archaeological and anthropological scholarship in the field of archaeoacoustics, the study of past sounds – the examination of the sonic understanding of the environment. Many of these studies are concerned primarily with deliberate sound creation through the manipulation of material culture, rather than the effect of sound itself (see collected essays in Scarre and Lawson 2006; Watson and Keating 1999). There are a few exceptions which examine the presence and effect of sound on the environment (King and Santiago 2011), and the soundscapes of sites as part of the experience of the space (Cocroft and Wilson 2006: 20–1). Sound recording has proved an effective means of accessing historical soundscapes. Notably, research on Stonehenge has examined the acoustic properties of the monument and its capacity to manipulate sound (Till 2011). Study of sound in this book draws on Steve Feld's conception of the idea of acoustemology, that is everyday sounds and how they affected one's experience of 'being in the world' (Feld and Brenneis 2004: 462). Analysis of the everyday sounds of the asylum can contribute to the broader picture of internal environment experience.

The historic sonic environment can be accessed through the material indicators and historical documentary evidence supporting the use and consideration of sound in the construction of lunatic asylums. Changes in the buildings over time, not to mention the difficulties in recreating a full-to-capacity lunatic asylum, make accurate recording of the sonic environment on the ground impossible, while it is not possible either to determine levels of past appreciation (Corbin 1995: 184). The material wealth of sound indicators and their presence in the historical record, however, make historical sound and its impact an accessible avenue of sensory study. Collaborative use of archaeological phenomenological approaches with more established methods (Hamilton *et al.* 2006: 31), such as historical sources, has proved a richer and less problematic avenue of research for lunatic asylums. This research will compare the historical documentary evidence with the material culture, in an attempt to determine the sensory concerns and safeguards of the architects and authors of reform literature.

Portable material culture from Irish and English asylums in the early nineteenth century has not been commonly retained by the institutions or by local heritage bodies, and apart from the buildings themselves, material remains are scarce. Some museum collections retain material from this period, such as small privately run mental health museums in Wakefield and Dublin. The survival of material remains varies from collection to collection, however, reliant on private donations and the discretion of the health services and developers. Portable material culture from the period is rare, but sometimes makes its way into local museum collections. The Stephen Beaumont Museum of Mental Health at Wakefield in England holds a significant amount of debris and material recovered from the Stanley Royd Mental Hospital (formerly the West Riding District Asylum) before demolition and development on the site. While heritage frameworks in England and Ireland are increasingly cognisant of the importance of retaining post-medieval and later historical materials from development-led excavations, the sheer volume of innocuous building material in these institutions means that the material is rarely retained. Buildings are extensively recorded by commercial archaeology units before demolition or redevelopment; examples of such include heritage assessments at the former Crooked Acres Hospital (a twentieth-century mental hospital) by ARCUS in 2008 (Cooper 2008), and the Victorian asylum, Bexley Hospital, by English Heritage in 1992 (Richardson 1992). For the purposes of this research, standing built heritage was photographed extensively, as access and permissions would permit, and the photographic record was supplemented with archaeological site reports, aerial photography, cartographic sources, and material culture where available.

Historical documentary sources form the core primary source material in this book. Historical records provide documentary evidence for management and practice in asylums, but they are also the most abundant material sources available for the study of historic lunatic asylums. The documentary record is a rich source of artefacts from the historical context in question (Wilkie 2006: 14). Like a platter or a ceramic bed pan, a ledger from an asylum office is an artefact as well as a useful documentary source. Documentary sources are employed as written texts and artefacts in this book. Extensive comparative analysis of material culture with historical documentary sources is necessary to gain a holistic picture of asylum life. The use of historical records in historical archaeologies is well established in the discipline. Though oft-misinterpreted as a disparaging comment on the inferiority of our discipline, Ivor Noël Hume's statement about archaeology as the 'handmaiden to history' (1964) referred to the potential for archaeologists, with our unique perspective on the material environment, to populate written records with real people, providing a voice to non-literate peoples through material remains. Rather than filling in gaps, archaeological and material approaches can uncover that which lies outside of the written record, such as human agency or subaltern voices. The discipline of historical archaeology has since been well established, with archaeologists employing the historical record to good effect in informing interpretation of material remains. This is particularly evident in later historical archaeologies where the extensive historical record of bureaucracy makes up a considerable portion of material remains. In many multidisciplinary assessments of the material culture of nineteenth-century asylums, however, historical records have been used extensively to inform research, yet without reference to the potential of these sources as artefacts in themselves. In order to maintain their basic bureaucratic processes, institutions used large ledgers, accounts, and letters, and these records represent the material record of administration and bureaucracy in the text they bear, their physicality, and the imperative of storage implied by their very survival into the present day.

The idea of the book or text as a physical artefact from which cultural processes and attitudes can be inferred is well established in literature studies and codicology (the study of books as material). Book history scholar D.F. McKenzie, in an assessment of the designation of a 'text', recalled the origins of the word in the Latin, *textere*, 'to weave' (2002: 29) as referring to material, as well as words. Archaeological approaches to graffiti address the consideration of text as material culture in an explicit way. John Schofield and Paul Graves-Brown have examined graffiti as both a textual and material source in their study of 6 Denmark Street in London, interpreting the graffiti therein as an expression of the volatile interpersonal relationships between members of punk culture in London in the 1970s (2011). Similarly, Katherine Giles and Melanie Giles's study of twentieth-century graffiti in rural farmhouses in the Yorkshire Wolds looked at graffiti as the material, as well as textual, indicator of routines and accounts of life experiences (2010). In the context of an historical institution, Eleanor Casella's examination of prisoner graffiti in Ireland relating to penal transportation emphasises the act of the inmate in creating graffiti. Casella paints a vivid picture of graffiti 'painstakingly carved, scratched or pecked into the fabric of the cell interior', emphasising the emotion involved in the creation of these artefacts, as well as the physical exertion (2005: 457–8). While patient graffiti is difficult to identify on redeveloped asylum walls, the written records compiled by clerks and doctors are not written without feeling. The compilation of text is part of the active (and emotional) taskscape of the asylum, through which human agents operate.

Beyond historical archaeology, the study of texts as artefacts is common. For example, medieval illuminated manuscripts are studied as both material and visual culture and given the well-known subject of most illuminated manuscripts (biblical transcriptions), they are arguably more useful as material and visual sources informing on the period in which they were composed than the text itself. Relevant for this study, as Chapter 3 will examine in more detail, is the study of illuminated manuscripts as physical, portable objects. A study of the Irish manuscript, the Book of Kells, looked at how the sourcing of extensive materials and exotic goods (200 calf skins for the vellum, and lapis lazuli for blue illuminations) evidence the importance of the book from its earliest days as an item of luxury (Rose 2011: 5). Historian Bernard Meehan has examined the vellum itself, suggesting that the monks responsible for the compilation and illumination of the book favoured a thick piece of vellum for pages of high illumination, demonstrating an active engagement with the physical arrangement of the book on the part of the illustrators (2009: 86). George Greenia has further argued that the creation of large volumes on which to transcribe and illuminate biblical texts in the Middle Ages attested to their status as totemic objects of power. A large book announced itself as a stage marker, signifying the status of the holder, binding them to their user groups (2005: 727). Large or expensively compiled books were carefully planned in their making and in their storage. In this book, the accounts ledger will be examined as an object of status and power, as well as a historical source.

Historical documentary research was carried out in archives and libraries, museums, hospitals, and using digitised online source material. The mass digitisation of rare books on the management of the insane and their publication online has aided comparative examination of these sources. Sources consulted included: plans and maps of lunatic asylum buildings and local areas; the minute books, accounts, and audits of individual asylums; government papers regarding lunatic asylum construction and administration; instructive texts on the construction and governance of the insane; and news media. Research on Irish asylums was occasionally hindered by a lack of surviving records; this is a problem commonly encountered by researchers in modern Irish history. In 1922, the Irish Public Records Office was destroyed. The office was housed at the Four Courts in Dublin and suffered heavy bombardment during the Irish Civil War by the forces of the Provisional Government while occupied by Irregular insurgents. Towards the end of the engagement, the Public Records Office was blown up from the inside by the occupiers. As a result, many public records – including the census data for almost every Irish county – suffered significant damage or were destroyed (Jackson 1999: 265–6). As such, there are many gaps in the documentary record. Demographic data and the content of government and census reports have been pieced together from parliamentary papers containing report summaries of commissions and committees. This material mainly comprises an overview of destroyed, yet detailed, accounts and records. As such, research in Ireland was heavily reliant on parliamentary reports and the preservation of asylum records or commissioner's reports onsite in the asylums themselves, as well as relevant correspondence from the Chief Secretary's Office, architectural plans, and government audits.

Management, space, administration, and the built environment

When they were constructed, asylums represented the physical manifestation of reform ideals, architectural principles, and innovative design approaches. The buildings underwent significant change during their tenure as public institutions and now present major challenges to local authorities and private developers as listed structures with problematic histories, linked in the popular imagination to narratives of abuse and confinement. Employing archaeological approaches to the built and material environment, as well as the historic documentary record, this book will address the built heritage of the historic lunatic asylum. Approaching the asylum and the built environment of insanity as archaeological artefacts and landscapes, this book will draw together archival source material, material culture, built heritage, and cartographic information to present a broad view of public lunatic asylums from the late-Georgian legislative frameworks which provided for their mass construction, to the Acts and changes in management and architectural practice which preceded the more widespread construction of the Victorian asylum system under the Commissioners for Lunacy. The legacy of these early decades of public *asylumdom* are key to understanding the built heritage and legacy of historic asylum buildings as they face massive redevelopment in the twenty-first century.

This book is organised into three thematic sections: asylum management, asylum administration, and movement through the asylum. The application of management and design practices outlined by lunacy reformers will be assessed in Chapter 2. In order to determine the extent to which reform principals were adopted and practised, spatial layout and design will be explored through the analysis of building plans and annual audits. Examination of management practice will highlight how the rhetoric of lunacy reform was applied at ground level, in the architecture and in management structures, taking into account the ongoing process of refining asylum management throughout the early nineteenth century. Chapter 3 will address the running of the institutions and the material culture of asylum administration. The spaces and processes of administration, as well as the materials implicated in bureaucratic process, inform on staff and patient hierarchies and the ways in which asylum spaces – interior and exterior – were actively employed in the running of the institutions. Internal staff and patient hierarchies are a central theme of Chapter 4, which will examine the spatial boundaries and pathways which determined the development of the asylum over time and led ultimately to a major design overhaul of the building type in the 1840s. The use of interior and exterior space informs on the extent to which reforms were incorporated into asylum architecture and management at ground level. Concluding with an overview of the archaeology of lunacy, the final Chapter 5 will address the ongoing issues surrounding the redevelopment and reuse of these still controversial sites, examining the historic communities which have grown around these institutions. This chapter will address the stigma associated with asylum buildings, in light of their (sometimes misunderstood) pasts.

2

Management

In order to facilitate the expansion of the century-old Maryborough District Lunatic Asylum buildings in 1933, architectural plans were drawn up for a set of glass verandas, one on either side of the building (Sheahan and Clery 1933). Though the building had been adapted and changed significantly since its construction, the 1933 plans indicate that the architect and the asylum authorities intended to maintain the symmetry of the building, consistent with every other addition to the front of the asylum since its construction. All additions to the Maryborough Asylum had kept the line of the original building, extending it laterally and eastwards as demand dictated, but never obscuring the west-facing facade. Architecturally, the Maryborough Asylum is a good example of an Irish provincial asylum built in the first half of the nineteenth century; it is also a good example of the extent to which these buildings were adapted significantly over time to cope with overcrowding, increased demand on services, and changes in patient management. At the Maryborough Asylum, as in other contemporaneous asylums, maintaining provision for equal numbers of men and women meant that the buildings developed almost symmetrically to either side of the original core structure; this continued throughout the nineteenth century and sometimes into the twentieth. The preoccupation with features like architectural symmetry and space among architects and asylum authorities alike sets asylums apart from other contemporaneous institutions like prisons or workhouses, which developed more organically as demand dictated. Symmetry, facade preservation, and the careful landscape planning required to maintain them illustrate the extent to which asylum architecture was almost an extension of the carefully ordered management regime within.

Some buildings eventually ran out of space and were abandoned entirely for newer asylums. Where the original building was constrained by geographical features or surrounding development, some local authorities opted to construct brand new facilities on greenfield sites which could be more easily adapted. The Dublin Union House of Industry is a good example of this. The institution was constructed north of the River Liffey, to the northwest of Dublin city centre in the 1770s: institutional support for the growing number of paupers in the rapidly expanding city. By 1820, demand on the services in the House of Industry had necessitated the spread of that institution into several separate hospitals, including a fever hospital, a children's asylum, a surgical hospital, and the Richmond District Lunatic Asylum. The need to accommodate multiple different classes of inmate in the House of Industry not only trumped the need for architectural symmetry, but stylistic and architectural continuity too. The hospitals of the Dublin House of Industry were a mixed bag of styles, ranging from classically inspired pediments and facades, to courtyard ranges that bore a stronger resemblance to small-scale industrial workshops than other workhouses of the period. It is not surprising, therefore, that when the asylum needed to expand its services in the 1850s, a greenfield site was chosen to the west, rather than construction on the already overcrowded asylum and workhouse sites.

The ideas and rhetoric which inspired the construction of asylums in the early nineteenth century will be juxtaposed with the built environment and the institution-specific needs which drove individual asylums to adapt their buildings in certain ways. Far from homogenous, asylums were highly specialised to their local populations. The material fabric of the buildings themselves evidences the individuality of local authorities in their approach to asylum building, and the varying interpretations of reform ideals such as moral management and non-restraint. Asylum architecture and the use of asylum buildings is frequently generalised; given the many commonalities – aesthetics, for example – between asylum buildings, it is easy to forget that asylums were a new kind of institution to many of the early architects. Where architects had experience of building hospitals or even lunatic wings or private asylums, the reformed public asylum presented new challenges, like patient classification according to the severity or manner of their insanity as well as their gender and class. As such, many architects and advising physicians took the opportunity to employ architectural features not commonly used in asylums and apply highly experimental designs. Unware of the demand which would be placed on public asylums, local and national authorities contributed varying sums to their construction. The result of this regional variation and experimentation was that early nineteenth-century asylums differed significantly from place to place and were as much a reflection of the architect's ideas and constraints as a practical application or venue for the ideals of asylum reformers.

The idea of moral management is often cited in the history of medicine as the driving force behind the reform of treatment for insanity and asylum management practice in the nineteenth century. The management of patients in a humane and caretaking manner – which reflected the ideas of asylum reformers like Samuel Tuke, William Sanders Hallaran, and non-restraint advocates like Edward Parker Charlesworth – was contingent upon the spaces in which management was practised. Archaeological approaches to lunatic asylums have compared instructions and guides on asylum construction and form with the remains of asylum buildings (see Piddock 2007). The influence of these instructions is evident in the built form of Victorian asylum buildings, including the classification of inmates, the provision of outdoor space, and adequate bathing facilities for the patient population. Many of these features were implemented in Georgian asylums first and influenced asylum reform authors like John Conolly in the compilation of their lists of instructions. Building on Susan Piddock's archaeologically focused analysis of asylum designs in the Victorian period, this chapter will explore the material application of the above-mentioned experimental ideas and trace the success and failures, as well as adaptations, of these designs over time.

Reform, management, and moral ideals

In the history of lunacy, the theorising and adoption of moral management in public and private lunatic asylums from the beginning of the nineteenth century is credited as a key turning point both in how the insane were treated in an institutional context, and how the idea of insanity was conceived of more broadly as a social problem, solvable with a modern solution. A more moral approach to the management of the mad defined what can be seen as a heroic phase of lunatic asylum reform in the late eighteenth- and early nineteenth-century, led by the ideas of men like Tuke, Pinel, and Charlesworth. This period of experimentation and early adoption of management practices is the usual preamble to histories of madness. Adoption of the broad range of ideas which made up moral management and non-restraint was a hard-won process for the reformers. This is partly because the idea of moral management is not easy to define and was not consistently codified by the large number of reformers who wrote about it.

Moral management does not refer simply to morality in the behavioural sense. The word 'moral', in the case of the late eighteenth-century lunatic asylum, referred to morality as an early modern social attitude, the outcome of a paternalistic drive towards a moral and improved society throughout the early modern period. The adoption of a moral approach to the treatment of the insane was ongoing from the late eighteenth century in many different forms, in asylums and hospitals in the British Isles, British colonies, North America, and continental Europe. This new approach to management was heavily influenced by the treatment of King George III by his physician Francis Willis. George III and his well-known madness raised public awareness and sympathy for the mad, particularly towards the second half of his sixty-year reign when his symptoms were manifestly too pronounced to be ignored or downplayed (Arnold 2008: 146). In 1788, the King's condition had deteriorated such that his own physicians were no longer up to the task of managing him, and Francis Willis was sent for on the recommendation of Lady Harcourt, Lady of the Bedchamber of the Queen, whose mother had been successfully treated by him (Macalpine and Hunter 1991: 51–3). He was a well-known physician based in Lincolnshire, who ran a madhouse out of his own home in Dunston and opened another in Stamford. Willis was also notable for propagating the idea that madness was curable (Parry-Jones 1972: 75–6). He was well known for employing moral authority and fear in his management method to subdue his patients. Willis was one of several mad doctors operating in the period who employed experimental techniques to treat the mad instead of resorting to manacles and isolation. One of these techniques, as described by historian Andrew Scull, was 'the eye': subduing a patient by startling and staring them down and applying the fullest moral extent of the supervisory gaze to cow them (1993: 69). Techniques like this demonstrate how mad doctors were already looking beyond physical restraint for more complex, psychological (moral) means of managing patients. Willis's methods were personal, one-to-one, and placed a level of trust in the patient to manage himself (Willis allowed the King a razor for shaving, for example) (Porter 2004: 162–3). Willis claimed that his management practice was influenced by William Battie, an English physician of the mid-eighteenth century and chief physician to St Luke's Hospital for Lunatics in London. Battie published an early treatise on the treatment of insanity (Battie 1758; Porter 2002: 103). His maxim was that 'management did more than medicine' in the case of madness. He was outspoken against the (often violent) treatment and confinement of patients at the public London asylum, Bethlem (Andrews et al. 1997: 276). His approach was highly influential, as it suggested that the mad could be cured, in a sense, by kind and patient treatment. This is the kind of language employed by successive writers on asylum reform. Two individuals heavily associated with the practical application of this moral approach to asylum reform were York-based asylum owner William Tuke and the French physician Philippe Pinel. Both men ran institutions: the Retreat and Bîcètre, respectively. Tuke founded his asylum, the Retreat, in reaction to the death of a patient after mistreatment in the York County Asylum. His new asylum was intended to be run along moral lines.

Pinel was a vocal advocate of the abolition of mechanical restraint. He was noted for releasing his patients from the chains binding them in favour of non-mechanical restraints such as straitjackets and leather muffs (Pinel 1806: 51–4; Thompson and Goldin 1975: 58; Yanni 2007: 24). This approach to abolishing coercion and reducing mechanical restraint was popular, but rarely successful. One of the few places that successfully implemented this system of moral management was the Lincoln City Asylum, under physician Edward Parker Charlesworth and surgeon Robert Gardiner Hill. Other asylums, encouraged by the writings of reformers like Pinel, attempted to replace mechanical restraint with other methods of managing patients. Cork City had an asylum, though it was not purpose built, overseen by asylum reformer William Saunders Hallaran. Hallaran operated as physician to the public asylum and designed a version of the 'circulating swing', a device originally devised by physician Joseph Mason Cox at the Fishponds private asylum near Bristol (Kelly 2008a: 82; Noll 2007: 203). The aim of the circulating swing was to revolve the agitated patient at a speed of up to 100 revolutions per minute. This, it was thought, would shock the patient into calmer, saner behaviour. The swing could also be used to subdue an unruly patient, as the rapid revolutions of the swing could cause patients to bleed from the nose and ears and occasionally induce unconsciousness (Ellis 1838: 228; Hallaran 1818: 90). The threat of use of the swing as a means of controlling or calming a patient may not be discounted. Circulating swings were popular in the early decades of the nineteenth century and used widely. William Ellis employed the use of a circulating swing at the West Riding District Asylum in Wakefield, apparently with success; but he pointed out in his 1838 treatise on insanity and treatment that use of the swing was a last resort and was only used under the careful supervision of the medical superintendent (1838: 227).

Under William Tuke, and later his grandson Samuel, moral management at the Retreat took the form of humane caretaking in a purpose-built institution, where the architecture was considered to be an active element of the treatment process. This included the provision of fresh air through openable and accessible windows, and open outdoor spaces where a patient could take exercise. The idea behind the Retreat was that ordered, sane design encouraged the maintenance of a sane environment within (Edington 2007: 86–7). The Retreat was designed by London-based architect John Bevans, and its construction overseen by local architect Peter Atkinson. The Retreat was arranged with a three-storey central block with sitting rooms and offices, flanked by two two-storey wings for patient bedrooms. The building was constructed of brick. The Retreat's arrangement of rooms in wings leading towards a central administration, a hidden utility block behind the main structure, and careful control of spaces had a significant impact on the ways in which asylum design developed. The design of the Retreat owes much to the rural, middle-class domestic dwellings familiar to the architects and William Tuke (Akehurst 2010: 89). Like the Tukes, Bevans was a Quaker, and had experience in constructing meeting houses; Bevans and Tuke have been credited with the design of the Retreat, while Atkinson is little known. Indeed, in her architectural history of the Retreat, Ann-Marie Akehurst has posited that Atkinson, as a non-Quaker, has been omitted from the historiography of the asylum (2010: 82). As such, the local character of the Retreat, as a Georgian dwelling in York, has been downplayed in favour of its impact as an architectural architype for moral management. For all of its fame and the central position it holds in the historiography of medicine, however, the Retreat was not, in itself, suitable for reproduction for public asylums. Bevans's son, James, though a noted and reputable architect with an interest in asylums, was himself rejected as the architect of at least two public asylums in Ireland and Wakefield. The arrangement of the Retreat was actively advocated as a model for a moral asylum by Samuel Tuke, whose writing on lunatic asylum management was a popular go-to for local authorities in the 1810s. In the mid-1810s, Tuke was called upon by the local magistrates of Wakefield to compile a list of instructions for architects in advance of the competition for the construction of the West Riding District Asylum, on the back of his reputation as an expert on the subject after publishing a description of the Retreat in 1813. Tuke provided detailed descriptions of the physical building, including features which ranged in detail from 'eight galleries' and 'a work room', to the overall separation of male and female patients, spatially, within the building (Tuke 1819). In seeking this expert advice, the local magistrates evidenced the widespread interest in constructing purpose-built asylums, in which moral management could be deployed from the outset.

The manager – occasionally referred to as the moral governor – was responsible for the everyday management of the asylum, usually in consultation with the visiting physician, with whom some managers had a sometimes fraught relationship. The position entailed overseeing the management and running of the asylum from within. The manager was responsible for the governance – moral or otherwise – of the asylum and was distinct from the physician as they were resident in the asylum. The duties of the manager required him to be actively involved in the day-to-day running of the institution. The manager at the Maryborough District Asylum, for example, was expected to inspect the male patients every evening, and to adhere to the recommendations of the physician for patient care (Jacob 1833: 54–5). On a practical, everyday level, though, the role was likely more nuanced, and encompassed staff, as well as patient, management. The manager was responsible for writing reports and checking accounts. Before the management of asylums was codified and refined in the middle of the nineteenth century, the practice of asylum management, and certainly the uptake on moral management in particular, was nuanced and varied between practitioners. Even in his treatment of George III, Willis deployed a mix of intimidation, threats, and moral boosting (Porter 2002: 103), as opposed to the regime of 'kindness and morality' as recommended at the York Retreat. As such, moral management and its employment was not a uniform or standard set of management techniques and is difficult to reduce to a generalised set of behaviours and rules. Equally, the role of the manager varied. Uptake of principles of moral management was selective and varied from asylum to asylum. Asylum architecture and the material control of the asylum's lived spaces was not enough to promote the adoption of moral treatment, but it was indicative of a general drive towards moral management, particularly those aspects of asylum architecture which were adopted well into the Victorian period.

Asylum planning and architectural design were codified towards the middle of the nineteenth century, following the 1845 Lunacy Act and the widespread construction of massive public asylums at county level in England and Wales, as well as Scotland and Ireland. John Conolly's influential book on asylum architecture, *The Construction and Governance of Lunatic Asylums and Hospitals for the Insane* (1847), is a notable contribution to the literature on ideal asylum architecture, as was his later work, *The Treatment of the Insane Without Mechanical Restraints* (1856). In his 1847 book, Conolly published lists and descriptions of features to be incorporated into an ideal asylum, drawing on the practice of moral management and non-restraint at the Middlesex County Asylum at Hanwell. The practical treatment of the insane is examined in more detail in his 1856 book. The Hanwell Asylum is an early example of the successful incorporation of principles of moral management into the running of a public asylum. Conolly's main thesis was similar to the writing of Tuke in the 1810s, in that classification and the careful division of space was central to the architecture of the ideal asylum. The building itself was to act as a guide for the rehabilitation of lunatics, an architectural instrument which would encourage saner behaviour among the patients. Patients were to be divided according to the severity and nature of their illness, their sex, and their class or status as fee-paying or public. Leisure and work quarters would also be separated from living spaces.

However, despite the popularity of the rhetoric of Tuke, Conolly, and other asylum reformers among local authorities, the managers of provincial asylums were sometimes frustrated by the rhetoric of reformers and thinkers who were not in the position of trying to run a public asylum on a day-to-day basis. Dr Charles Corsellis, the manager of the West Riding District Asylum in 1844, remarked on the lack of practicability of some of the more theoretical notions of his contemporaries, particularly in light of the massive overcrowding which necessitated a programme of expansion at the Wakefield Asylum almost as soon as it was constructed. He says of reform writers that:

> the most pernicious effects have resulted, from theoretical and visionary notions of the condition and wants of the insane, and from an attempt to grasp an imaginary perfection, whilst the dictates of common sense, and the results of sound practical experience, are overlooked. (Corsellis 1844: 22)

Corsellis's frustration is reasonable. He was probably also lashing out at his rival, the visiting physician to the Wakefield Asylum Dr Caleb Crowther; their fraught relationship will be discussed later. As the individual responsible for the everyday management and running of his asylum, Corsellis was (understandably) frustrated by the attempts of men who had no connection to his institution to dictate how asylums should be ideally run. His remarks can be read as a statement of discontent with the flaws in how the Wakefield Asylum was designed, i.e. its architectural mechanics. The Wakefield Asylum is credited as the first purpose-built asylum for the reception of the public, designed purposefully for the moral management and non-restraint of patients (Smith 2007: 54). The West Riding Asylum was directly affected by the advent of reform rhetoric and writing on moral management, as the instructions for the architects were penned by Tuke himself, who also advised the magistrates. Tuke's recommendations and instructions were distributed to prospective architects, alongside a Request for Proposals in 1814. The specifications were in fact published along with an introduction by Tuke and the successful plans of the architects, Watson and Pritchett, in a volume in 1819. Reform was part of the very material fabric of the Wakefield Asylum from the outset.

As well as the ideas behind the management of patients, the ideal asylum designs and specifications were not always adopted, or even advocated, by those involved in individual asylum design. For example, the Board of General Control in Ireland – who were responsible for the planning of provincial asylums in Ireland in 1817 – found themselves at odds with the government in Ireland, despite the government's interest in establishing improved institutions for public confinement and welfare. The undersecretary to the Lord Lieutenant of Ireland at the time was Robert Peel (who would be prime minister of the United Kingdom in the

1830s and 1840s), who tried to persuade the board to adapt a disused eighteenth-century pre-reform gaol in Roscommon for the purpose of a provincial lunatic asylum as a cost saving measure, rather than constructing a new building (National Archives of Ireland Commissioners for General Control: OPW 999/784, 19.09.17). It was the architect, Francis Johnston, who argued against this as the building could not be adapted so as to be in any way morally beneficial for the patients. Moral management was a key concern for the Board of General Control when they were building their provincial asylums. During the design process, Johnston expressed multiple concerns, including over public perception of how asylums operated and how his designs would be employed. He was concerned, for instance, about the popular notion that frantic and unruly lunatics were kept in basement cells (National Archives of Ireland Chief Secretary's Office: CSO/RP/1818/390/6; National Archives of Ireland Commissioners for General Control: OPW 999/784, 23–5). His concerns were not unfounded, as the popular legacy of the eighteenth-century asylum as prison-like in character was not improved by Johnston's designs, either. Johnston's most commonly constructed design was the Class Two K-shaped provincial asylum for 100 patients, which was criticised heavily in *The Irish Builder* in 1867 as a therapeutic instrument with the character of a prison (Fogerty 1867: 39–40). The moral environment of the asylum remained a concern for critics and architects well into the Victorian period.

The role of the moral manager was clearly laid out and defined in didactic publications which appeared periodically, penned by key figures in asylum reform rhetoric. Conolly himself outlined their role (1847: 133), while in Ireland the role of the manager was laid out clearly in the early minutes of the reports of the Irish Commissioners of Lunacy, prior to and following the establishment of the first Irish provincial asylum at Armagh in 1825 (National Archives of Ireland Commissioners for General Control: OPW 999/784, 275; 349). However, the manager (sometimes the director) was a relatively new role in the wider context of institutional management of the insane. Previously, the treatment and management of patients in asylums had been ultimately overseen by a physician. The Monro family of physicians of Bethlem Asylum are a particularly illustrative example of how physicians – indeed, several generations of them of the same family – came to dominate the ways in which patients were treated. In the damning evidence which asylum physician Thomas Monro gave to the Committee on Madhouses in England in 1815, which ultimately led to his dismissal from Bethlem, he outlines the various means by which madness was treated at the asylum, stating that he was the head of medical affairs there (First Report 1815: 93). Though casting blame for ill treatment at the door of other men responsible for the asylum, such as the apothecary John Haslam, his testimony reads as that of a man of the highest authority within the institution. In that report, prior to the widespread construction of public asylums at provincial level, the physician was presented as the most senior authority in patient affairs. In such a context, therefore, the introduction of the position of manager was sure to ruffle the feathers of local physicians throughout the British Isles when public asylums opened their doors in the 1810s. As the proprietors of private asylums themselves, the visiting physicians can be forgiven for assuming a degree of authority.

Physician dissatisfaction can be found throughout the didactic literature on the treatment of the insane in the nineteenth century. In his own treatise on lunacy, Maryborough-based physician John Jacob wrote an account of the duties of managers which held more than a few veiled criticisms of the manager of his own District Lunatic Asylum (1833: 43–4). The position of the manager at the Maryborough District Asylum was taken by William Abbott in 1833. Abbot was responsible for the practical running of the asylum and the implementation of moral management and non-restraint, which was eventually taken up in 1842 (The National Archives of the United Kingdom Audits of Maryborough: AO 19/48/14). Prior to this, mechanical restraint was still employed and manacles and straps were used to restrain patients (The National Archives of the United Kingdom Commissioners for Auditing: AO 2/68; 69; 70). Abbot himself was impressed with the effectiveness of non-mechanical restraint (The National Archives of the United Kingdom Audits for Maryborough: AO 19/48/14); strong dresses (strait jackets or other garments designed to restrict movement) were put to good use in 1842. Abbot's reaction to their effectiveness demonstrates the scepticism among provincial asylum managers about the practicality of some of the ideas for reform and moral management which were being espoused in the literature.

Non-restraint as a method for managing patients was popular in the rhetoric and instructive writing which preceded and coincided with the construction of public asylums. In his damning testimony to the Committee on Madhouses in England 1815, Monro stated that the use of mechanical restraint was not fit for 'gentlemen', but suitable for use on paupers, not least given the issues in staffing a public asylum to the same extent as a private asylum in order to maintain order when restraints were not applied (First Report 1815: 95; Arnold 2008: 174). The outcome of Monro's testimony to the Committee indicates that his opinion was no longer that which was widely held by the government authorities overseeing the construction and management of asylums. Monro's testimony gave further weight to the popular opinion that Bethlem, as it had been, could not continue. The situation at Bethlem became apparent after a patient, James William Norris, died following his release from the Asylum where he had suffered a sustained period of apparent maltreatment. Norris had been confined to a harness for over a decade, preventing easy movement, and the testimony of Monro and Haslam with regards to his treatment was enough to damn them in the eyes of the Committee (Porter 2004: 131). Norris's harness was described in the Committee report in detail:

> a stout iron ring was riveted round his neck, from which a short chain passed to a ring made to slide upwards or downwards on an upright massive iron bar, more than six feet high, inserted into the wall. Round his body a strong iron bar about two inches wide was riveted; on each side of the bar was a circular projection, which being fashioned to and enclosing each of his arms, pinioned them close to his sides. This waist bar was secured by two similar bars which, passing over his shoulders, were riveted to the waist bar both before and behind. The iron ring round his neck was connected to the bars on his shoulders, by a double link. From each of these bars another short chain passed to the ring on the upright iron bar. (First Report 1815: 12)

Norris communicated his distress at such a confinement to the Committee representatives, apparently lucidly, from his cell. Rather than being left to his confinement, Norris informed on the active malicious intent of the keepers at Bethlem, stating that a chain connected him with a keeper next door, who could pull it and move Norris at will. Among his visitors was an artist who sketched his sad situation and an engraving of the treatment of Norris made by George Cruickshank was published widely in the popular press (Porter 2004: 131). This image, though made before Bethlem was relocated to the new asylum at St George's Fields, was frequently featured in the press for the following two decades (Cross 2012: 26) as a visual representation of the sorry state of public asylums. The popularity of the image, and the impact it had – alongside the description of his harness – on the Committee and the general public, shows that there was wide interest in an alternative to restraint in public asylums.

New ideas about non-restraint were entertained where they could be put into practice. The method had the most marked success at the Lincoln City Asylum, which opened to patients in 1820 and was managed from the outset with a view towards moral treatment, in spirit if not always in practice. The asylum was managed by a board of governors, among them local physician Edward Parker Charlesworth. In the 1820s, Charlesworth advocated increasing regulation of the asylum at Lincoln, promoting the admission of visitors to allay any fears of maltreatment and, most significantly, the abolition of restraint for the patients. After the death of a patient in 1828 by strangulation on his bed restraints, Charlesworth's ideas gained momentum (Smith 1995: 57). Along with the efforts of asylum surgeon, Robert Gardiner Hill, mechanical restraint was abolished at the Lincoln Asylum by the end of the 1830s. Hill himself went on to pen a history of the abolition of mechanical restraint (1857). Success at Lincoln had a considerable influence on moral management as an effective treatment technique. However, the question of who exactly would manage the asylum was the source of widespread debate, and occasionally conflict.

The position of the moral manager was subject to scepticism and attack from critics, specifically medical men associated with asylums, from the time each asylum opened. That the asylum was under the primary control of the moral manager rather than the physician was a particular point of contention. Charlesworth and the director of the Lincoln Asylum, Thomas Fisher, had a tumultuous relationship, leading to Fisher's eventual dismissal. Mental health historian Leonard Smith has suggested that some local opinion at the time held that Fisher had intended to provoke Charlesworth into a duel (Smith 1995: 57), so fractured was their relationship. At the Maryborough Asylum, John Jacob, as a physician himself, promoted the expansion of the role of the physician in local asylums, and suggested that the moral manager had a responsibility to work under the direction and authority of the visiting physician, presumably due to their greater medical expertise. In his book, Jacob attacked the Maryborough Asylum manager, Abbot, over the value of his position and asserted that the physician be afforded more power over the day-to-day running of the asylum. With the consent of the governing authorities in Dublin, overall authority over the Maryborough Asylum was passed from Abbot to Jacob in 1834 (Grimsley-Smith 2011: 48). Jacob's ideas were published by an anonymous source in the *British Medical Journal* in 1839. Mental health historian Arthur Williamson has suggested that the anonymous author was Jacob's own brother, as the ideas espoused there were not widespread, but rather helped by a limited and select group of physicians in Ireland (Williamson 1992: 557). One of Jacob's concerns was the level of education held by a manager responsible for the moral management of an institution. He was, in this regard, likely supported by men such as the physician of the Richmond Lunatic Asylum in Dublin, Dr Jackson, who regarded the management of the first Irish provincial asylum at Armagh under its manager Thomas Jackson as being 'practiced from a book' and expressed concerns about the importance of a good temper and manner in a moral manager (Williamson 1976: 113–14).

In England, this same conflict was also being played out in provincial asylums. At the Wakefield Asylum, the visiting physician Dr

Crowther complained of being 'thwarted' by the manager, William Ellis, and later came into conflict with Ellis's successor, Corsellis, over how the institution was to be run (Bolton 1928: 591; Marland 1987: 321). Crowther published (apparently against the wishes of his family) a book of observations on the running of madhouses and expressed concern over the position of the moral manager in general. Instead, he advocated the appointment of a medical manager, who could be supported by the visiting physician (1838: 40–2). Where physicians were generally only connected to public asylums in a visiting capacity, many lived in their own private institutions. Writing on the construction and governance of asylums in 1847, Hanwell physician John Conolly expressed his frustration in relation to architects who, he stated, did not like to consult with the medical men who lived in the asylums and knew best the needs of patients (1847: 6). He blames this recalcitrance for the significant variations in asylum design and plan. Under moral management, the managers usually lived in the asylum and thus overtook the physician as the main point of contact for the outside world. As such, the conflict went beyond medical and managerial; the conflict between manager and doctor was as much about the control of space as it was about patients. In the medical profession in the early nineteenth century, appointment to a hospital was an important career move for physicians, and this kind of association helped to bolster their reputation (Geary 2004: 124). The creation of a new role in the moral manager may have been seen as a usurpation of a role or position in authority coveted by local physicians, who saw the asylums as their professional domain.

Despite these frequent conflicts between the men in charge of asylums, a 'moral' approach to the treatment of patients emerged as the most popular aspect of reform rhetoric in the early nineteenth century. A moral style of management was among those features of the asylum looked for by the Inspectors General of Asylums in Ireland, for example. In 1839, the Inspectors expressed their satisfaction with the moral character of the provincial asylums constructed in Ireland and referred in their report to both the management of the patients and asylum buildings (Fogerty 1867: 39–40). When his treatise on the construction and management of lunatic asylums was published eight years later, Conolly wrote moral management into the centre of the reformed asylum, as he envisioned it (1847; Piddock 2009: 189–90). However, moral treatment was not without its critics. Crowther, for instance, claimed that the Wakefield Asylum manager William Ellis, who would later manage the Hanwell Asylum which had been so influential to Conolly, had employed 'fallacies and tactics' to obscure the number of cures at his asylum. Crowther claimed that cure rates at the Wakefield Asylum were less than Ellis claimed in his reports (1838: 30). In light of Crowther's animosity towards the Wakefield Asylum management, though, his claim must be treated with some caution.

There were architectural requirements for the effective use of non-restraint and moral management according to the publications of the period, written by reformers like Tuke, physicians such as Conolly, Crowther, and Jacob, and asylum architects Johnston and Bevans. The built environment was considered to be an essential mechanism for conditioning behaviour. However, the practical requirements of maintaining and managing these spaces was not always clear, either from the literature or the plans. The reformed asylums, though built to be 'therapeutic instrument[s]' (Fogerty 1867: 39), frequently made for unaccommodating dwelling places, and the wear and tear of everyday use took its toll. Due to the materials with which they were constructed and the financial constraints on their running, asylums frequently succumbed to problems such as overcrowding, poor ventilation, and bad lighting.

The people who inhabited and moved about the asylum on a daily basis – the staff and patients – engaged with it in different ways: as a workplace, a temporary living space, a place of incarceration, and even as a home. For the architects of reformed asylums, the asylum as 'home' was one of their primary concerns. This is reflected in the preoccupation in architects' notes, as well as reform writing on asylum architecture, with the 'domestic' interior space of the asylum, for the benefit of patients. From the early nineteenth century, asylum interiors were intended to reflect the principles of moral management; an interior which was recognisably domestic, rather than institutional, would reduce the punitive tone of the architecture and provide inhabitants with a degree of comfort, within which environment they could presumably get better. At the Wakefield Asylum in 1844, Corsellis noted that it was designed to afford patients the 'comforts of home'. Conolly devoted much space in his treatise to the interior environment of the public lunatic asylum, which clearly influenced later decorative leaning in asylums after the 1840s. Conolly advocated a clean, comfortable space, in which to promote sleep and comfort for the patient (1847: 20). This aspect of the reformed asylum carried into the end of the nineteenth century, when public asylum interiors increasingly came to ape the style of a middle-class home (Coleborne 2010: 30–1; Guyatt 2004: 49).

Asylum buildings were constructed with the intention of housing, as well as treating, people. Patient experiences of asylums varied by individual, by institution, and by country, so it is not possible to ascertain – at least empirically – if patients considered asylums to be 'homes' in an emotional sense. The architectural arrangement of the buildings and their interior environments were certainly geared, at least initially, towards a domestic space, but this was mitigated by the degree of control and spatial management which was necessary in an asylum to maintain patient classification, discipline, and security. Most patients undoubtedly had some form of emotional relationship with the asylums in which they lived, whether fond or otherwise. Corsellis asserts that the Wakefield Asylum was considered with some level of affection among former patients, if the frequency with which former patients expressed a desire to visit their former asylum is any indication (1832: 7). Later in the nineteenth century, Wakefield Asylum director James Crichton-Browne records the practice again (Ellis 2001: 86). The rootedness of the asylum within memory as a prominent place of personal experience and growth was likely reinforced by the permanency of the architecture, while the emotional connection forged by patients was undoubtedly linked to the nature of their experiences there. Management of patients in a moral manner was more likely to foster a positive memory of the place. As such, the legacy of the asylum among the communities of patients of staff who interacted with them was intrinsically bound up in the success or effective execution of humane treatment and moral management.

Patient behaviour and staff duties

The practice of moral management on an everyday basis required the complicity of all parties to the principles of the ethos, and the adherence of those parties to the careful rules of the institution in which this was to be enacted. Much of the scholarship on the history of medicine, and particularly the didactic and summary texts composed during the nineteenth century, focuses on the role and activities of the asylum managers and physicians as the primary actors in the running of an asylum. General and support staff members are not strongly represented in the documentary evidence for asylums in the early nineteenth century, beyond occasional lists of staff names and their salaries. Keepers and nurses, laundresses, kitchen staff, and maintenance workers, on whose positions the everyday operation of the asylum hinged, are usually relegated to broad generalisations and anonymous job titles (Veis 2011: 52). The absence of these figures from the official narratives of asylums, rather than indicating their absence or inefficacy, shows that, as a group and barring exceptional or notorious individuals, these people carried out their duties with a relative degree of success. The contemporaneous (early to mid-nineteenth-century) literature on the roles and duties of keepers and asylum workers is very specific (see, for examples, Browne 1991; Conolly 1847: 105–19; Crowther 1838: 119; Ellis 1838: 272–30; Jacob 1833: 60–3; Tuke 1813: 145–9). However, given the frequency with which staff member behaviour and activity appears in both the didactic literature and primary source material, compliance with these directives was an ongoing, if small-scale, difficulty in public asylums.

Keepers – sometimes referred to as attendants – and nurses (if they were women) were the staff category who came into contact with patients most often. When keepers are mentioned in the primary and secondary literature on lunatic asylums, they were generally referred to in terms of their role as disciplinarians, as enforcers of moral management at the lowest level. A few more-notorious examples appear in individual asylum reports, government inquiries, or the popular press for their abuse of power, such as the 'three villains' of 1810s Bethlem Asylum: Blackburn, Rodbird, and Allen. These three were alleged to have neglected and abused patients to such an extent that several patients died under their supervision (Arnold 2008: 175). Problematically, these cases of abuse and violence are more notable in the historical record, and there are few first-person accounts (unsurprisingly) of keepers and nurses carrying out their daily tasks. It is therefore difficult to access the daily lives of keepers and nurses and their duties. Instead, accounts of what keepers and nurses ought to have been, and cases in which they were certainly not as they should have been, are the most telling primary sources for what the duties of the keeper or nurse were as the ground-level representative of moral management and the new asylum system.

Keepers and nurses, as noted, are rarely mentioned in the historical record in any great detail. Where they are referred to, sources often allude to keepers and nurses in terms of their physical presence, and their role as representatives of the institutional ethos or social ideology. Keepers and nurses, as the individuals most frequently associated with dispensing treatment on a daily basis, or with enacting disciplinary action when patients were acting out, have come to represent a shorthand for the institutional framework of the asylum in secondary literature. Australian historian Lee-Ann Monk argues, for example, that male keepers in Australian asylums in the Victorian period reinforced masculine gender dominance in the asylum, through the authority inherent in their position and their assertion of patient control through physical action. Thus, keepers asserted their masculinity among other keepers, as well as over the patients (Monk 2003: 70–1). In the same volume on Australian asylums and madness, Dolly MacKinnon includes the activity of keepers and nurses in the soundscape of asylums, as they were expected to use bells and whistles in the management of patients (2003: 76). I have built on MacKinnon's points regarding soundscapes, arguing that the possession and use of keys in the asylum created institutional soundscapes which were sometimes contrary to the moral management of patients (Fennelly 2014: 420). Sociologist Lindsay Prior asserted that hierarchy in the nineteenth-century asylum was reflected in the space afforded to individuals and staff categories, so that keepers had less space than their supervisors (the manager or matron) (1988: 106). The low position of the keeper or nurse within the asylum authority was indicative of the moral authority asserted by the manager and physician. Despite this, effective moral management of the asylum lay in the ability of these staff members to carry out their duties in an effective and moral way.

When the first reformed public asylums were constructed in England and Ireland in the early nineteenth century, the activities and habits of keepers and nurses were a cause for much anxiety to reformers and hospital managers. The type of person suited to the job, and even the requirements of the job, differed from institution to institution. Even the job title differed between different asylums and commentators, with some preferring keepers to attendants, for example. In his history of mental health nursing, Peter Nolan likened the term 'keeper' in asylums to that of keepers of animals and interpreted the uptake of the term 'attendant' after 1845 to indicate a more humanitarian approach to care (1993: 6). Titles steadily came to reflect an increasingly moral outlook in asylum management as the role was standardised and the concerns of the early nineteenth century overcome. The problem of sourcing responsible, sober staff was explored in several venues, with few solutions beyond the hiring of more, and better vetted, staff to relieve strain. In his book on the care and management of the insane, John Conolly pointed out that the selection of keepers and nurses was an under-explored subject in the wider discussion about asylum reform. He raised several concerns which reflect the state of public asylums in Conolly's own experience, such as rapid staff turnaround as a source of disruption for the patients, and the selection of keepers and nurses (attendants) without consulting the medical superintendent (1847: 83–5). In his annual reports on the Wakefield Asylum, Charles Corsellis recorded hiring more keepers in the early 1840s in order to reduce the workload on those already employed there (1842: 8). The (once lauded) architecture, he stated in his reports, was a hindrance to the work of the keepers. Corsellis blamed the keeper's difficulties in carrying out their jobs to the best of their ability on the size of the institution and the consequent problems encountered in supervising patients (1844: 5). Among the problems with keepers and nurses in the asylums were the frequent instances of their behaving adversely towards patients.

Keepers and nurses were generally local men or women who lived outside the asylum. Public asylums in the early nineteenth century were beset by many problems, not least the overcrowding of accommodation (discussed later in this chapter), and a high ratio of patients to staff – as discussed by physician and reformer W.A.F. Browne in his lectures on what asylums were, are, and could be (1837: 147). Keepers and nurses worked under the authority of the manager and matron. Their job was the supervision and superintendence of patients on a daily basis. There were no formal qualifications for keepers and nurses; for male keepers, physical strength and stamina were among the desirable attributes in candidates (Smith 1988: 306). Until 1885, there was no formal standard handbook for keepers and nurses that laid out the duties and behaviours of the job. The *Handbook for Attendants on the Insane* (Campbell Clark *et al.* 1885) was published at the end of the nineteenth century (Nolan 1993: 63). The 'Red Book', as this handbook became known, standardised the role of the keeper and nurse, and some institutions published their own rules and guidelines in addition to these. The County Council of Surrey, for example, published their own abbreviated Red Book of rules in 1929, which included a brief run-down of the ethos and aims of the hospitals in the county (1929). Prior to these publications, however, the role was selectively interpreted as each institution required.

In lieu of any formal training of asylum keepers and nurses, the job was carried out by men and women from different backgrounds. As most staff members were not subject to disciplinary action, the most that remains of these people in the historical record is their name, usually next to a wage figure in an account book. As such, it is difficult to know what brought most of them to the asylum for employment. What has been written about keepers and nurses, usually by physicians and commentators on insanity in the early nineteenth century, is telling of the social class to which most belonged. Given their manner of writing about the keepers and nurses, the physicians and commentators who wrote about their duties saw themselves in a higher social class. Among the instructions for the behaviour of keepers and nurses was advice on their manners, the use of appropriate (and inappropriate) language around the patients, and the importance of abstinence from smoking at work (Conolly 1847: 114; Jacob 1833: 62). In his treatise on public asylums in the 1830s (informed heavily by his own experience at the Wakefield Asylum), physician Caleb Crowther recommended that the army would provide an ideal source of male keeper for the asylums of the aristocracy (1838: 119). Crowther's idea indicates his awareness of the importance of discipline and respect for hierarchy in the qualities of a keeper.

It is probable that former military men were attracted to the position of keeper in government-run lunatic asylums, particularly during the economic recession which followed the Napoleonic Wars. The influx of thousands of able-bodied and idle young men onto the British and Irish labour market after demobilisation in 1815 posed a significant problem for the British economy. The situation was further exacerbated by a sharp decline in some of the industries which could have supported these men – such as iron working, which had been supplying the war (Brown 2003: 352; White 1957: 148–9). Several memorials were made to the Lord Lieutenant of Ireland in the late 1810s and early 1820s from former members of various regiments or their family members asking to be considered for employment. One from a woman, the wife of a former lieutenant of the 90th Regiment of Foot, then confined to the Richmond Lunatic Asylum, sought consideration for employment as housekeeper at the Richmond Penitentiary (National Archives of Ireland Chief Secretary's Office: CSORP/RP/1820/367). Another, from a surgeon who had served in the Peninsular War, asked to be considered for appointment to one of the provincial lunatic asylums under construction in 1821 (Chief Secretary's Office Registered Papers 1821). The men who came out of the army in the 1810s were disciplined and strong, a key quality in male keepers as previously mentioned. Therefore, veterans of the wars, their wives who may have been used to the discipline and rigours of military service, or even the disciplined industrial workers and skilled artisans who found themselves out of work after the war, would be suited to the role.

Before the system was more uniformly organised under the Lunacy Commission in the 1840s, each asylum had their own rules for behaviour and conduct among patients and staff members. The rules of each asylum reflected the moral ethos and ideology under which influence the reformed lunatic asylums were established. The following quoted section, dating to 1816, details the expected conduct of patients at the Richmond Lunatic Asylum. The language of the rules reflects the origins of the asylum as an ancillary institution to the House of Industry, while the threat of bodily confinement indicates that the principals of non-restraint were secondary to the maintenance of order in the asylum, even while the moral management of the asylum was a priority.

> Rules for the Conduct of Patients, sanctioned by the mangers to be hung in Day Rooms
> Whoever shall break windows, or is in other respects mischievous shall have the arms secured.
> Whoever shall offer violence to any person shall have the arms secured and shall be subjected to solitary confinement.
> Whoever uses profane, scurrilous or indecent language shall be degraded to the Frantic Ward.
> The managers of the asylums whose views are amply secured by the conduct of the moral manager, are averse to the adoption of any severe measures which are however indispensable for the general security in case of wilful opposition and which will therefore be steadily enforced.
> (National Archives of Ireland: Richmond District Lunatic Asylum Minute Books 1: 2.9.1816)

These rules were to be posted on black boards in the day rooms, and reflect the expectations on keepers to maintain order, as well as expectations of patient conduct. That such a collection of rules was compiled in the first place indicates that managers and overseers of the asylum and House of Industry were concerned with discipline, likely reflecting previous breakdowns in order in the House of Industry next door. It is unclear if these boards were ever actually mounted on the walls but, if they were, their limited efficacy is reflected in an entry in the Richmond Asylum minute books in 1817, repeating the order for the rules to be painted on boards and mounted in day rooms.

The usefulness of these boards was dependent upon the ability of patients and staff alike to understand them. In the early nineteenth century, roughly half of the adult population was expected to be illiterate. In England, average adult literacy rates grew from 50 to 58 percent between 1754 and 1837, with lower rates (between 40 and 50 percent) in the major cities and industrial centres (Stephens 1987: 5–8). This data is not conclusive, however, as these percentages are drawn from research on marriage certificates, reflecting the number of people who could write their own names rather than those who could easily read a book – or a board of rules (Hewitt 2000: 64; Vincent 1993: 16–17). Novelist Charles Dickens portrayed the widespread problem of partial literacy in the personage of Joe Gargery, the brother-in-law and father figure to Pip, the protagonist in *Great Expectations*. Set between 1812 and 1830, Gargery is shown to recognise his own name easily enough but is largely illiterate otherwise (Dickens 1861). Though adult literacy rose through the nineteenth century due to the establishment of the National School system in England and Wales, and later in Ireland, literacy rates among older adults remained low. As such, only half of the adults, patients, keepers or nurses employed in the asylum could have been expected to be able to read the rule boards at the Richmond Asylum in full. The display of writing, given the low level of literacy that could be expected among the patients, keepers, and nurses, suggests that literacy itself was employed as a tool of authority. The rule boards were actively employed in the imposition of a social hierarchy, a superiority suggested through the use of written words. The literacy of the asylum and House of Industry managers, the expectation of a knowledge of the rules on the part of the keepers and nurses, and their responsibility to impose these on the behaviour of the patients, communicates the social hierarchy of the asylum as one based on competence through literacy and education.

A low level of literacy among pauper patients, and probably keepers and nurses too, meant that the display of rules likely served another purpose beyond informing the reader, and that was to communicate the expectations of the institution authorities through the material display of this artefact of order and authority. The board was an instrument with which keepers could subdue patients, a representation of the limits of behaviour which the asylum could tolerate in patients, as well as a display of the ethos of the asylum. The entry in the Richmond Asylum minute books in 1817 advises that the rules are for the 'ordering' of patient conduct, suggesting that the boards were intended to be used by keepers as a point of reference. Maintaining order in the asylum was essential to situating the asylum more broadly within the framework of order and improvement which was sweeping across England and Ireland at this point. This period of mass institutionalisation in England and Ireland, what has been referred to by historian Michel Foucault as the Great Confinement, coincided and was heavily informed by a movement towards improving and ordering public spaces and imbuing the streetscape with a spirit of obedience. The improvement of civic spaces like Sackville Street in Dublin, or the imposition of grid patterns in new city centres like the Edinburgh New Town, were part of this movement. Archaeological studies of urban landscapes and neo-classical architecture in the early modern period have correlated the creation of improved cityscapes with the creation of elite and non-elite landscapes (Matthews and Palus 2007: 230). Social division and classification were written into the improved city, creating designated spaces for movement, for dwelling, commerce and recreation, and institutions like prisons, workhouses, and asylums for those who could not adequately contribute to the working life of the increasingly industrial land- and cityscape. The Richmond House of Correction, south of the River Liffey in Dublin (also designed by public works architect Francis Johnston), mounted an inscription of the motto of the city of Dublin above their gateway which captured the ethos of moral planning and civic improvement: *Obientia Civium Urbis Felicitus* – 'Obedient Citizens make a Happy City'. Coupled with the inscription over the House of Correction doorway, 'Cease to do evil, learn to do well', the moral weight inherent in public institutions like the House of Correction, the House of Industry, and even the Richmond Asylum, was clearly and authoritatively communicated through architecture and material display.

The behaviour of all staff was carefully monitored in the new asylums. As well as keepers and nurses, other support staff were expected to report to the manager and matron and contribute to the overall moral, as well as industrious, life of the institution. Each asylum had a number of utilities – including kitchens, brewhouses, bakehouses, farms, and laundries – to support the asylum from within. This was an early articulation of what sociologist Erving Goffman came to call a 'total institution', where all of the needs of everyday life were catered for in-house (Goffman 1976). In common with the patients, each of these support staff had carefully defined rules governing their behaviour. As the asylums grew in size and capacity, these duties became more refined and closely monitored. By the end of the nineteenth century, for example, laundresses in British and Irish asylums were expected to record all of the details of their working week into a laundry book, which was presented to the medical superintendent every week for inspection (Burdett 1891: 228). A reiteration of the duties of one of these support roles may accompany an entry in asylum minute books outlining an individual's failure to carry out these duties, or their actions against the moral character of the institution. When Richmond Asylum laundress Eliza Long and her colleague Mary Anne Nicholson were found to be supplementing their wage packets with contributions from the male keepers, the manager called for a cessation of the practice and increased their wages (National Archives of Ireland: Richmond District Lunatic Asylum Minute Book 10: 26.4.1859). Though the women were likely doing nothing more harmful than taking on extra laundry for the single men they worked with (since they were not dismissed, any illicit practice can be discounted), such close fraternisation was not encouraged. A non-regulated and unrecorded activity was not considered to have a place within the asylum. However, evidence of resistance to this rigorous control of space and behaviour is not uncommon in the historical and archaeological record.

Resistance to or the transgression of socially acceptable behaviours in an institutional context was not confined to the patients. Archaeological approaches to subversive resistance among staff and inmates in institutional contexts uncovered networks or communities of collective insubordination, evidenced by the smuggling in and distribution of illicit objects and substances (Casella 2007: 71), or the creation and maintenance of distinctive identities and social roles among inmates (Mytum 2013: 181). In the case of working asylums, many of which are still in use as hospitals or redeveloped as apartment buildings or offices, it is not always possible to identify these material indicators of transgression. However, it is still possible to identify collective resistance in the recorded activities of individuals or groups of general and support staff. By posing archaeological questions about material indicators of resistance in the written historical record, the underside of the strict institutional codes of behaviours can be inferred. While not always explicitly recorded, resistance to the rigours of institutional life among the lower levels of the staff hierarchy can be inferred from the frequent revising and restating of the duties and rules for behaviour in the historical record. When the Richmond Asylum manager called for the rules for patients to be painted and mounted on boards in the day rooms for a second time, it is clear that these rules were not being followed. Among the staff, a community of peers developed that could not be regulated or managed by the asylum. The active community of staff suggested by the case of Long and Nicholson at the Richmond Asylum contravened the hierarchy of the asylum. By socialising, staff acted outside of their accepted behaviours, in active resistance to the asylum. In all of the detailed treatises and descriptions on moral management, asylum architecture, and the careful control of space and behaviours published in the early and mid-nineteenth century, the human agent within the asylum is discounted. The contrary actions and activities of individuals and groups are not taken into account in the planning process. It is for this reason that the public asylums quickly ran into difficulties early on, when the careful plans of the architects and reformers were systematically undone by their inability to control the sheer number of people who sought 'asylum'.

Overcrowding: building for ideas, building for demand

The asylum, as a setting for the application of innovative reformed management practices and a therapeutic instrument in itself, was only as effective as its material environment. Factors such as continuous use, weathering, light or lack thereof, and temperature impacted the efficacy of the rooms and airing yards, however well appointed. A major contributing factor in asylum efficacy was population. Plans for early nineteenth-century asylums are clear about the number of patients they can accommodate; for example, in his initial studies for the provincial asylums to be constructed in Ireland, Francis Johnston clearly states that his radial-plan asylums were to house 100 patients (St Patrick's Hospital Archive Plan No. 2: F/8). As such, the everyday operation of the asylum, and thus effective management of patients, was hampered by the admission of more patients than could be reasonably housed within. Among the reasons for asylum overcrowding were flaws in management practice, the suitability of buildings to cater for the wider locale, and external economic factors, such as famine or war. Most asylums responded to these circumstances by expanding, rapidly, sometimes within just a few years of operation.

The cure of the insane was foremost in the minds of asylum reformers, and the readmission of repeat patients or the admission of incurable patients was not recommended. Tuke and other reformers foresaw the problems which over-admission might cause, hindering the operation of the public asylums. Cure was central to the moral management thesis (Field 1994: 3), and central to the mission of asylums if they were to maintain patient turnover and stay in operation. As such, asylum designers favoured an asylum design which was more suited to a general infirmary or hospital than to the dedicated long-term reception, treatment, and accommodation of refractory (violent or acute) patients (Walsh 1997: 162). Despite these efforts, most asylums were operating over capacity from the time they opened.

Samuel Tuke held that 200 was the maximum number of patients who could be reasonably accommodated in a public asylum to allow for the adequate practice of moral styles of management (Smith 1999: 81). Tuke was an advocate of the potential for asylums to cure patients (1813: 132–3), but he was aware of the potential problems posed by overcrowding; his own private asylum, the Retreat, was built to accommodate thirty patients, but housed fifty by the time Tuke wrote his descriptions of the institution in 1813. Indeed, he suggests that the Retreat not be held up as any model for asylum architecture (1813: 104). As such, the recommendations which Tuke makes for building public asylums are more telling of popular approaches to implementing moral management in purpose-built asylums than practice at the Retreat.

Tuke advised on the material features and architecture of the Wakefield Asylum at the invitation of the local magistrates. Among other recommendations, Tuke advised that the asylum be constructed to allow for the expansion of the buildings, if necessary (expansion from an original occupancy limit of 150, to 200). Available space was divided evenly between male and female patients. As such, the number of places for patients at the Wakefield Asylum was informed by a therapeutic and management ideal, rather than by the real demands on the system locally. The industrialisation of nearby cities like Leeds and Sheffield in the early decades of the nineteenth century saw the population of west and south Yorkshire bloom rapidly, as migrants from the rural hinterlands flocked to the cities for work. Wakefield was a market town, standing amid towns and villages which quickly became associated with coal mining. As one of the major commercial centres in West Yorkshire, the population of the town expanded accordingly, and in 1821 had a population of 10,764 (Baines 1822); the West Riding had an overall population of c. 625,000 in 1811, rising rapidly to 801,000 in 1821. Despite this increasing demographic, a government survey in 1801 indicated that there were just 424 lunatic poor residing in the West Riding, housed in a variety of institutions, including workhouses and prisons (Report from the Select Committee Appointed to Enquire into the State of Lunatics 1808). Tuke himself estimated more than 650 lunatic poor in the 1810s (1819: 6), but despite this demand outside of the asylum system, still recommended places for a maximum of 200 patients. These negligibly low estimates were corroborated by evidence presented to the Select Committee appointed to consider the better regulation of madhouses in 1816, and first published by the Royal College of Physicians, where it was stated that the institutionalised lunatic population in all counties outside of London between 1810 and 1815 was roughly twice that of the city itself (1816: 79). London, it seemed, had a far more pressing problem with lunatics than the rest of England; the institutionalised lunatic population of London was likely a more accurate reflection of the number of institutions for confinement in the city itself, rather than an accurate representation of the potential demographic for provincial asylums. The private patient population in 1819 was recorded as 2545, reflecting a more realistic estimate that was, surprisingly, not taken into account when public asylum population figures were calculated (A Return of the Number of Houses for the Reception of Lunatics 1819: 7).

Tuke's reasoning for such a small number of patients at the Wakefield Asylum, and for the magistrates' acquiescence, likely lies in the faith of reformers in the ability of asylums to cure their patients and thus guarantee a high turnover of admission cases. The cost of housing a larger number of patients must have also been taken into account. The extensive expansion of the Wakefield Asylum buildings in the decades immediately following its opening indicates failings in both the system of management and the architecture to provide a necessarily rapid turnover of patients to maintain the asylum as it was. Indeed, the issues raised by overcrowding meant that parts of the building not initially intended for patient use at all, such as the front basement (initially intended for the use of lay labourers), was given over to housing increasing numbers of patients (Corsellis 1832: 4). The operation of the asylum as a therapeutic environment was thus interrupted when spaces unsuitable for the application of moral management were employed for patient housing. The asylum did respond to these problems in rapid fashion. A new wing was constructed at the Wakefield Asylum in 1831 (just over a decade after the original asylum building opened for patients) for the reception of seventy additional male patients. This wing was followed ten years later by a corresponding wing for female patients (Corsellis 1844: 5), implying that there was higher demand for accommodation for male patients than female patients, at least initially.

Gender classification was central to reformed asylum design. This fundamental means of patient classification was carried through every iteration of asylum design in the nineteenth and twentieth centuries; early twentieth-century asylum architect G.T. Hine noted in his description of British asylum architecture in 1901 that the division of asylum buildings by gender was a natural given (1901: 197). German asylum reformer and psychiatrist Maximilian Jacobi even went so far as to suggest that all facilities in asylums be doubled up, ensuring that male and female patients would never mix (1841: 26). However, while separate baths and yards were reasonably feasible, Jacobi's suggestion was expensive when extended to include other utilities. In any case, the separation of patients by gender was a fundamental aspect of the reformed asylum and facilitated in the asylum buildings by architectural symmetry. Yet, the strict, symmetrical division of patients to dedicated parts of the asylum building may have further irritated the problem of overcrowding. Demand for space and accommodation was not, it is clear from the records, gender equivalent. In 1832, Dr Corsellis noted in his reports on the Wakefield Asylum that 784 male patients and 745 female patients had been accommodated in the asylum since it opened. Closer scrutiny of the figures reveals that, of the patients no longer resident in the asylum, only 373 male patients had actually been discharged. This is in contrast to 442 female discharges. Corsellis also noted that male patient death rates in the asylum were higher than female patients, at 270 male patients to 175 female patients (1832: 10–11). Male patients appeared to have been accommodated in the Wakefield Asylum longer than female patients, while female patients were more commonly admitted on a casual or short-term basis. This explains why additional accommodation for male patients was constructed before expansion of the female wing. This difference in admission rates may be linked to the differences between male and female patients diagnoses. Cases of 'hysteria' and 'melancholia' were more commonly diagnosed among female patients, as well as conditions associated with pregnancy and childbirth (Arnold 2008: 217; Levine-Clark 2004: 134). These diagnoses relate to acute and frequently short-term illnesses, likely related to stress, brought on by poverty and lack of financial independence, or to perinatal depression or illness. As such, higher discharge rates among female patients are not surprising. That this dichotomy in admission trends was not taken into account in the planning of the asylums, however, certainly is.

Symmetry and architectural style must have played a significant part in how asylums were designed, at least as much if not more than admission or discharge data. What asylum designers and the magistrates or governors who supported them thought about how the buildings would function when expected to cater for the demands of the population is something of a mystery, given the problems which overcrowding caused in asylums in the early to mid-nineteenth century. The design for the block-plan Richmond Lunatic Asylum (Figure 2.1) indicates that patient classification along social and gender lines was more important than the needs of the mad who, when the asylum was being designed and built, were inadequately housed next door in the House of Industry. As such, the number of people, as well as their classification needs, could already be surmised from the available sample of potential patients. From the time it opened, the asylum was very careful of the number of incurable patients admitted, demonstrating an awareness of the potential for overcrowding if all classifications of patient were admitted immediately. Correspondence between the asylum physician Dr Alexander Jackson and the House of Industry next door, in 1816, records that extra space was available in the asylum for twenty female patients, which could be filled by incurable lunatics from the House of Industry (National Archives of Ireland: Richmond District Lunatic Asylum Minute Book 1: 2.09.1816). Despite the best efforts of Dr Jackson and the governors of the asylum, however, the careful division of space at the Richmond Asylum was soon disrupted by the need to maintain gender classification in outdoor space and by the limitations of the building itself. The asylum was carefully planned so that fee-paying male and female patients could be housed in separate quarters from the pauper class and had access to dedicated outdoor space (Irish Architectural Archive Murray Collection: 0092/ 046–0411). This kind of social classification was intended to attract the kind of patient whose contributions could support the asylum. The inhibitions of Francis Johnston's enclosed courtyards on the flow of fresh air and sunlight (Fogerty 1867: 40), however, meant that the careful ordering of internal and external space was interrupted in 1819 by the appropriation of the front garden for female patients and the yard behind the laundry for all male patients, regardless of class (National Archives of Ireland: Richmond District Lunatic Asylum Minute Book 1: 14.05.1819). The difficulties surrounding issues with overcrowding and low patient turnover, and the agitation resulting from constant construction work on and around the asylum buildings over a decade and a half, suggest that practical concerns such as accommodation were behind the decisions of management to delay the implementation of reformed systems – such as non-restraint – in any meaningful way, until 1838.

    Until practical matters such as accommodation, access, and recreation could be addressed, the management were not in a position to experiment with ideology and reformed management practices. The solution at the Wakefield Asylum was to add to the new building, rather than employing other institutional buildings to ease the burden on the asylum. This dedication to the form of the asylum as a standalone institution attests to the importance of a purpose-built asylum to the ideology of reform. The reformed management practices espoused by physicians and the government in their reports and enquiries were intended to be implemented in spaces designed for that purpose. In Ireland, this mission was less on the part of the government advisors than the public works architect who had been appointed to explore options for asylums at provincial level. In 1817, the Irish Board of General Control appointed public works architect Francis Johnston to oversee the construction of provincial asylums. Johnston's experience of asylum

Management 59

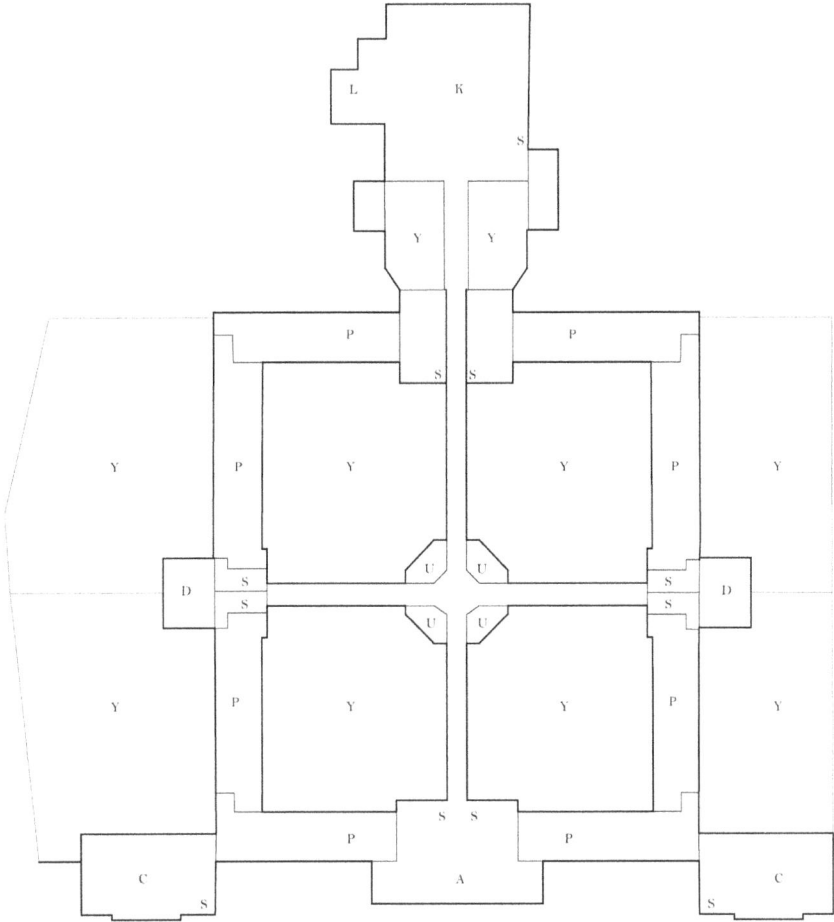

Figure 2.1 Richmond District Lunatic Asylum ground floor (1814). Administration (A), Convalescent rooms (C), Day Rooms (D), Kitchen (K), Laundry (L), Patient Rooms (P), Stairs (S), Utilities (U) and Yard (Y).

design was limited to assistance on the eighteenth-century expansion of accommodations at the private St Patrick's Hospital, and the outdated courtyard-style Richmond Lunatic Asylum. The Richmond Asylum had been purposefully constructed for lunatics, to relieve pressure on the House of Industry, but was closer in material and style to the House of Industry next door and the radial-plan prison to the north. In designing asylums to be constructed as institutions in their own right in the Irish provinces, Johnston looked elsewhere for inspiration. His objection to the reuse of Roscommon Gaol indicates that he was aware of what was certainly unsuitable and demonstrates Johnston's knowledge of the need for the proper classification of patients in moral management. In addition, Johnston appears to have been aware of the ideology and reform rhetoric surrounding asylum design elsewhere, as he argued in the case of Roscommon that the building could not accommodate patients 'with any degree of comfort or much prospect of relief' (National Archives of Ireland Commissioners for General Control: OPW 999/784, 17.09.17).

In his diaries, later in life, Johnston underplayed his own contribution as a public works architect to the streetscape of Dublin. In a short list of the buildings he planned and executed, he included the Richmond Asylum, but appears to dismiss his many other contributions (including, presumably, his work on planning the as-yet unbuilt provincial asylums) as 'many minor buildings not worth mentioning' (National Library of Ireland: MS2722, 1820). As well as being an obvious choice of appointment, being at that time the public works architect, Johnston was also stylistically suited to the construction of institutional buildings. Indeed, his austere and utilitarian aesthetic style in the 1810s and 1820s, what his biographer and architectural historian Edward McParland has called his 'penitentiary style', suited the mission of his institutions for carceral confinement (Boyd 2016: 9). Johnston's naturally understated and unassuming aesthetic style meant that in some cases he was even asked to modify his designs to reflect a grander vision; architectural historian Richard Butler has compared Johnston's built and unbuilt designs for the provincial courthouse in Armagh, demonstrating the increasing stylisation of the building in the planning process (Butler 2015: 115–20). As such, Johnston's asylums are not, in context, very austere or institutional-looking. Given that Johnston applied this style in many of his buildings, such as the General Post Office, in provincial courthouses and other municipal buildings, and in domestic architecture, his asylum facade designs were relatively innocuous in the Irish streetscape.

Johnston's asylums, like their English counterparts, were constructed for 100 or 150 patients, depending on the design. Unlike the designs of his rival for the job of planning the provincial Irish asylums, architect and asylum commentator James Bevans, Johnston's plan was intended from the outset for expansion or even reduction. Bevans's proposed design, £6000 more expensive than Johnston's, was a radial plan and self-contained, in many ways the very height of fashion for the purpose-built reformed asylum. Johnston's 150-patient asylums could be expanded to accommodate 172 patients (or reduced to accommodate 128) without additional building work (National Archives of Ireland Commissioners for General Control: OPW 999/784, 23–5). Johnston went so far as to provide estimates for high and low patient numbers. Given his knowledge of the necessary classification and comfort essential for moral management, Johnston was probably also aware of the conviction of reformers that moral management could cure madness and thus ensure a frequent turnover of patients. As such, his designs were limited by the idea of cure, by the number of patients who could be accommodated, and by the broad classification of patients according to gender, social class, and diagnosis facilitated by symmetrical architecture. It is not surprising that Johnston's designs, when put into practice as working asylums, were almost immediately rendered unsuitable due to overcrowding and demand. By 1843, there were 2028 lunatics housed in Irish asylums (most designed according to Johnston's specifications), in a system meant to support just 1220 (Finnane 1981: 34).

Overcrowding and the over-prescription of interior and exterior asylum space according to ideal admission and discharge rates, rather than realistic demand, resulted in the massive expansion of these early purpose-built asylums within just a few decades. Private asylums were opening at a rapid rate in England and Ireland to cater for fee-paying patients who could afford to look beyond the inflated public asylum systems. The idea that public asylums could be supported by voluntary donations and public subscription had not come to pass; in many ways, this was not surprising. This same failure in encouraging public interest and donations had been behind the widespread construction of private madhouses in the early modern period (Foucault 2006: 40). Given the demand for accommodation, public asylums in Ireland and England between the 1820s and 1840s were more or less constantly under construction and expansion. The construction work would have interfered significantly with the carefully planned sonic environment (discussed in more detail in Chapter 4), as well as access to interior and outdoor space as intended. To attract fee-paying patients, managers had to maintain certain standards in their asylum buildings so that the public asylum could be considered an attractive alternative to a private institution (Smith 2007: 123). Under the circumstances, and given the necessity for extensive building works, such standards could not have been maintained. In addition, the therapeutic mechanism of the asylum building was disrupted. The construction of the female wing at the Wakefield Asylum, for instance, interrupted the carefully laid mechanisms for surveillance and spatial management inherent in the building plans, as designed by the architects Watson and Pritchett and advocated by Samuel Tuke (Figure 2.2). The asylum, as a lived-in building and working institution, was typified by the case of the Wakefield Asylum. The expansion of that building to accommodate increasing demand signifies the degree to which the asylum was physically adapted according to the needs of the patients and the management, and not according to an ideal to maintain the optimal asylum plan. Despite this, the Wakefield Asylum was and is still frequently written about, in

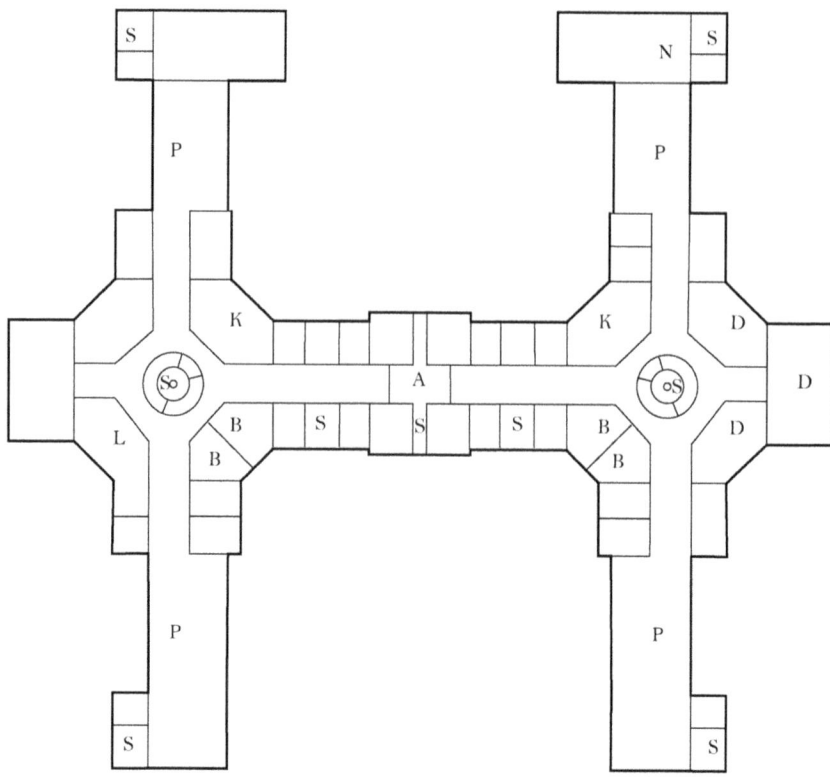

Figure 2.2 West Riding District Lunatic Asylum plans by Watson and Pritchett (1819). Administration (A), Baths (B), Day Rooms (D), Kitchen (K), Laundry (L), Noisy Patient Rooms (N), Patient Rooms (P), Stairs (S).

contemporaneous literature and the historiography, in model terms – as a talisman for early nineteenth-century moral architecture (see, for examples, Edington 2007; Jacob 1833; Jacobi 1841). In practical terms, the original plan of the Wakefield Asylum lasted just a decade, when it was deemed unsuitable for demand and adapted accordingly. While architecture is frequently written about as essential to the mission of moral management, commentators rarely look beyond the original plans to how the buildings were adapted to respond to crises.

The solution to overcrowding at public asylums in England and Ireland was, in most cases, the massive expansion of the asylum buildings, and thus a disruption of the intended spatial ordering of the interior and exterior space. There are a few exceptions. For example, the Lincoln Asylum was so put upon for space, and in need of such extensive expansion to cater to demand, that the construction of an entirely new asylum was deemed the only solution. In 1857, the building which had been the

Lincoln Asylum became a private institution, while public patients were admitted instead to a larger, purpose-built asylum on the city fringes, at Bracebridge Heath. A similar approach was taken at the Richmond Lunatic Asylum in Dublin when the accommodation requirements on the asylum outgrew the site itself. Beginning with the construction of an infirmary and chapel on open land to the west of the asylum site in 1849 (designed by the firm of Johnston's nephew and protégé William Murray), the Richmond Lunatic Asylum expanded into new buildings at different times, as demand required, throughout the nineteenth and twentieth centuries. The original asylum building became the Female House (for female patients only) in the 1890s, and a corridor-plan asylum was constructed for both male and female patients on the new asylum site to the west in the same decade. This new asylum, like the inspiration for the original Richmond Lunatic Asylum, was designed according to the style of private residences in the period (Taylor 1991: 54).

Plans of the Richmond Lunatic Asylum, the 'Female House', in 1899 indicate that the interior of the asylum had been altered significantly from Johnston's original plan in the eighty-five years since its initial construction (National Archives of Ireland Plans of Clonmel Asylum: OPW 5HC/4/799). Where Johnston had designed the three-storey building in a hollow square, with a single-storey cruciform corridor dividing the interior yard into four separate courtyards, by the end of the nineteenth century the cruciform corridor had been demolished to make way for a large dining hall which occupied the central space, bisecting it and leaving two enclosed yards to either side. The original plans for the Richmond Lunatic Asylum had indicated that the front yards be designated for male or female patients of superior social class, with rear yards set aside for male or female patients of the pauper class (Irish Architectural Archive Murray Collection: 0092/046–0411). The destruction of the divide between the social classes indicates that social segregation in the asylum ceased to be a consideration for these yards. The rear yards, converted in the 1810s for the use of male patients, had all been built on with utilities by the end of the nineteenth century. In addition to these changes, the internal plan of the building was altered. Open-plan wards took the place of the original arrangement of individual bedrooms, allowing for the accommodation of larger numbers of patients. The irrevocable and thorough reconstruction of the interior and exterior spaces of Johnston's first public asylum evidence the scale of demand on the asylum building to necessitate such change, as well as changes in thinking about what asylums should be like during the nineteenth century.

Changes and alterations to existing asylum buildings were echoed in the Irish provinces. Johnston's provincial asylum plans had been adapted and implemented by William Murray after Johnston's death in 1829 and were constructed with little variance across the country in the 1820s and 1830s. The first Irish provincial asylums began admitting patients in the 1820s. The provincial asylums at Armagh (1826), Londonderry (1828), and Belfast (1829) were similar in elevation, if not in plan, to Johnston's provincial asylum drafts from the 1810s (St Patrick's Hospital Archive Plan No. 2: F/8). While Johnston's early plans were cruciform, these were K-shaped, and built to accommodate 100 patients. Two cruciform asylums were constructed, at Limerick (1827) and Ballinasloe (1833), these for up to 150 patients. Though enclosed by yard walls, these asylums were situated on new and unenclosed sites. Learning perhaps from his mistakes at the Richmond Lunatic Asylum, Johnston's new asylums were sited where they could be expanded, on the outskirts of towns and cities, close enough to be convenient yet remote enough for privacy. This reflects how asylum buildings were conceived of in the years immediately after the first dedicated reform pauper asylums were built and situated. The Middlesex Asylum constructed at Hanwell north of London in 1831 came to represent this second generation of reformed asylums. In his book on the treatment and management of lunatics, Middlesex Asylum manager William Ellis was clear about the importance of a 'healthy situation' (1838: 268). Ellis, who had previously served as the manager for the Wakefield Asylum, advocated the choice of site and situation over the necessity of economy for both the bodily health and mental comfort of the patients, as well as the convenience of land for patient occupation. In choosing an asylum site conducive to fresh air and space, Ellis suggests that some of the effects of massing large numbers of people together, notably disease and illness, might be circumvented (1838: 271). As Ellis pointed out in his book, inadequate space for asylums led to higher mortality rates. External factors such as illness and epidemics, as well as socio-economic crises in the 1830s and 1840s in both England and Ireland, further exacerbated the issue of low patient turnover and increased overcrowding.

The first major expansions to accommodation in the provincial asylums in Ireland coincided with a period of significant economic upheaval and crisis: the Great Famine. Successive years of blight on the potato crop, the staple food of most of the Irish population in the 1840s, led to half a decade of privation. A laissez-faire approach to the crisis on the part of central government led to significant loss of life, as well as massive rural depopulation due to emigration, disease, and starvation (Woodham-Smith 1962: 411). Migration from the countryside into major towns and cities was common; the famine and the privations of its aftermath also led to mass emigration from Ireland to England and the

United States. The famine had an impact on the supply of food to public asylums, as well as placing great strain on the asylum system in general. The main staple of the public asylum patient's diet in Ireland was the potato. A typical diet consisted of oatmeal for breakfast, potatoes with either buttermilk or soup for dinner, and a supper of white bread. Male patients could expect up to 4 lbs (1.8 kg) of potatoes every day, while female patients could be served 3.5 lbs (1.5 kg). This menu was served at the Maryborough District Asylum in 1844 as standard (The National Archives of the United Kingdom Audits for Maryborough: AP 19/48/14). Potatoes were a convenient source of cheap food for public asylums. Culturally, they provided a continuity of diet for pauper patients, especially those who had been transferred from local workhouses where the diet was similar. Potatoes were a cheap source of nutrition and ideal for supporting a day's labour (Davies 1994: 549; Ó Gráda 1999: 18). They were conveniently widely and consistently grown in rural Ireland, all year round, and could be grown in large numbers in limited space (Sabine 1823: 265). Indeed, consistent use of the same small plots of land exhausted the soil and contributed to the spread of the blight. Continued blight over successive years made the small plots of land typically farmed by the rural Irish farmer useless for feeding their own families, much less for supplying public asylums with excess.

The audits of a provincial asylum like the Maryborough Asylum reflect increasing difficultly from the early 1840s in sourcing potatoes to satisfy demand. The asylum did increase its provision for patients at this time; in 1846, local builder Pat McEvoy was employed to adapt the former straw and workrooms at the asylums for the accommodation of thirty additional patients (The National Archives of the United Kingdom Audits of Maryborough: AO 18/48/14). However, the scale of difficulty is not consistent with an increase of just thirty patients. The staple food at Maryborough changed abruptly in 1847 to bread (The National Archives of the United Kingdom Audits of Maryborough: AO 19/48/14: March–May 1847). Indian corn meal, rice, oatmeal, and soup also appeared in increasing quantities, just as the supply of potatoes dwindled. Institutional diets in England were significantly different, suggesting that the dominance of the potato in the Irish institutional diet was as much cultural as economic. Of the six model menus distributed to provincial workhouses in England by the Poor Law Commission in 1835, only four included potatoes. Indeed, where they were included, the portion sizes were considerably smaller than those in Ireland, just 0.5–0.75 lbs (0.2–0.3 kg) per day (Higginbotham 2008: 51–5). Irish asylum expenditure on food jumped sharply, and very suddenly, between 1845 and 1847; from £968 to £2054 at Maryborough Asylum, and £2044 to £2657 at Richmond Asylum, for example. Figure 2.3 illustrates a sharp

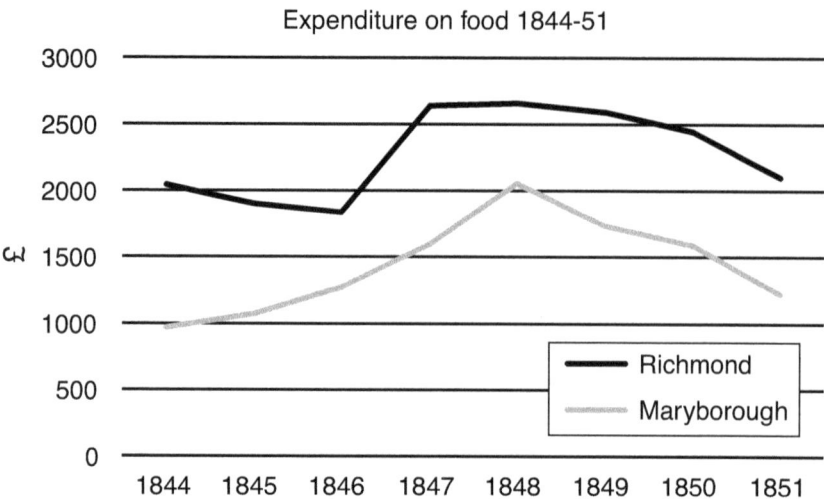

Figure 2.3 Expenditure on food in two Irish asylums from 1844–51, spanning the peak years of the Great Famine.

peak in food expenditure at the two Irish asylums in 1847. This peak subsides gradually over the following years, but expenditure on food remained higher than pre-famine levels as the crop recovered.

The increased expenditure incurred by Irish asylums, workhouses, and other public institutions, necessitated by the change from potatoes to bread, meant that the food deteriorated significantly in quality. Nutrition-related diseases, such as scurvy, increased (Crossman 2006, 20). In his bioarchaeological evaluation of the Kilkenny Union Workhouse for this period, archaeologist Jonny Geber remarked that the high proportion of individuals affected by deficiency-related and infectious diseases at the site studied suggested that the malnourished inmates of the workhouse were more susceptible to diseases like cholera and typhus, endemic in institutional populations (2015: 185). The Irish Famine demonstrated the extent to which public asylums had become ingrained in the social geography of poverty. The burden of public relief for famine was passed from centralised government to the newly established Poor Law system during the crisis, exacerbating the already strained efforts of the large public institutions (Ó Gráda 1993: 108). Where there were no Poor Law workhouses to which people could turn, the burden of relief fell to what institutions were local. There was no workhouse at Maryborough during this period; the two workhouses located nearby, at Abbeyleix (14 km away) and Mountmellick (10 km away) were strained and overcrowded (O'Connor 1992: 178). The infirmary and the gaol at Maryborough had in the past picked up some of the burden of institutional care for the rural population outside of the town, such as during an outbreak of cholera in the town in the 1830s (National Archives of Ireland Cholera Papers: 2/440/9). A spike in the patient population coupled with a very low discharge rate at the Maryborough Asylum during the famine suggests that the asylum was contributing to the institutional management of the poor during this period of crisis (Report on the District, Local, and Private Lunatic Asylums in Ireland 1846).

The impact of the famine on the already overtaxed and overpopulated provincial asylum system was considerable, and the dramatic reform of the asylum system in Ireland, as well as England, in this period was necessary to respond to these difficulties. The increasing number of admissions and instances of overcrowding which preceded the rapid expansion of the provincial asylum system in Ireland may have been exacerbated by the famine. Those who were born or were very young during the 1840s in Ireland may have been impacted by the trauma of the famine, and thus the patient population was swelled (Grimsley-Smith 2012: 11). Indeed, starvation-induced or -aggravated mental illness was recorded in Britain in the case of pauper lunatics (Kelly 2004: 54–5; Showalter 1980: 162; Skae 1863: 318), so this must have also been occurring in Ireland in the aftermath of the famine. Mismanagement of this period of significant crisis and privation in Ireland thus may have inadvertently led to an increased burden on the state in both England and Ireland in the long term, given the impact of starvation and displacement on the mental health of the Irish people, into the second half of the nineteenth century.

Managing the moral asylum

Moral management, as espoused and implemented by the managers, physicians, and architects of lunatic asylums in Ireland and England in the first decades of the nineteenth century, was not a singular idea. Rather, moral management was a broad set of practices which included the abolition of mechanical restraint, the kind and humane treatment of the insane, and the implementation of behaviours conducive to an institution inspired by the middle-class home. Materially, the ideas of moral management manifested in the architecture of the public lunatic asylum. With only a few examples of the building type to which they could aspire, architects experimented with different building styles and sought innovative solutions to the ideas for perfect management practices posited by reformers and physicians. The lofty ideas of these men were tested when set against the demands of a public asylum system. The economic constraints of constructing asylums for the pauper class, particularly during the economic crises of the 1810s, meant that the ideas of moral management were not taken up in any uniform way. It is for this reason that asylums of this period vary considerably in style; indeed, the experimentation involved in early asylum design is the reason for many original asylum buildings' designation as historic structures in the twenty-first century, while later additions have been demolished.

Within the buildings themselves, the system of management in asylums which placed lay managers rather than medical men atop the asylum hierarchy meant that interpersonal and professional tension between asylum managers and local physicians was widespread. The implementation of such a rigorous system of management while also trialling the experimental architecture of the new reformed asylum exasperated the new public asylums almost immediately on their establishment and resulted in an overtaxed and inconsistent system of provincial asylums. Rapid overcrowding and the necessary expansion of asylum buildings from the outset confirms the inefficacy of moral management and a lack of consistent practice. Furthermore, low cure numbers and high admission rates attest to the inadequacy of provision and the limitations of moral management by itself, at least on a large scale. These failures led to an overhaul of the whole system in the 1840s, beginning with the Lunacy Act in 1845 and the establishment of the Commissioners for Lunacy.

3

Administration

William Farrell was in his twenties during the uprising in Ireland in 1798. Living in the south-east, an area of particular agitation, Farrell witnessed the unrest in his native Carlow and became a reluctant participant in an event which led ultimately to the hanging of eleven men in the town. His memoirs of the event, *Carlow in '98*, were published posthumously in 1949, edited by Irish academic Roger McHugh. The memoirs were written between 1835 and 1845 with all of the benefit of hindsight and no small degree of what McHugh referred to as 'tedious' moralising. By his time of writing, when he was into his sixties and seventies, Farrell was the newly installed gate lodge keeper at the Carlow District Lunatic Asylum, which opened in 1832. His job afforded him the free time to compose his memoirs, and he occupied the gate lodge at the asylum until his death.

Farrell is a singular figure in the historiography of the Carlow District Asylum, and in Irish asylum history more generally, in that his is a rare instance of a named gate lodge keeper outside of the context of asylum records or census data. Farrell was one of the support staff – along with clerks, laundresses, and maintenance staff – whose role was intrinsic to the running of the institution and who are yet underrepresented in the historiography of the history of medicine. Similarly, while the official records and accounts of public lunatic asylums are largely the domain of the reforming physicians and the radical managers, and are focused to a lesser extent on the patients, the individuals behind the composition of this record – the book-keeper or the clerk – are rarely explored in any detail. Support staff rarely appear outside of wage lists, despite occupying a key role in the processes which made the asylum work as an institution, producing the bulk of the material remnants of the asylum (the historical record), and engaging daily with the carefully planned geographies of the institutions themselves. Accounts of disciplinary action are frequently the only mention of the individual actions of support staff. These individuals rarely impacted the rhetoric on patient treatment, asylum management, and the architectural arrangement which dominated much of the didactic literature on insanity in the early nineteenth century, and as such their contribution to the successes and failures of experimental systems for treatment has been overshadowed by the role of doctors and managers. Support staff remain relatively anonymous.

This chapter will explore the role of support staff in developing, maintaining, and recording processes in the early asylum. It looks at how the asylum was actively and materially run, through the implementation, maintenance, and adaptation of administration and bureaucracy. The idea of hierarchy within the asylum will be examined, with a focus on the actions and processes which went into maintaining that hierarchy on the ground level, between staff and patient, staff and staff, and staff and public. Bureaucratic control and the effective practice of administrative process by all elements of the asylum hierarchy was essential to the maintenance of the status quo. The hierarchy of the asylum differed from that of other contemporaneous institutions, however, and each individual asylum operated their own form of administrative bureaucracy. The administration of asylums was codified and centralised under the 1845 Lunacy Acts, but these took some time to come into effect. This chapter will look at the operational systems of management and classification in the lunatic asylum among staff and patients at ground level and examine the material culture of bureaucratic process and the input of the civic government on asylum construction and running. Where the last chapter looked at how innovative management and designs implemented in the wake of government-level reform in the way madness was managed influenced the way the asylum developed over time, this chapter will shift focus to the ground-level systems and processes which were adapted and modified to be accommodated in the buildings as they were. Finally, asylum foundation, administration, and overall governance will be examined within a national context, as an institutional response to the consolidation of the state in both England and Ireland. With reference to English regional examples, but with particular emphasis on Irish asylums in the aftermath of Union with the United Kingdom in 1801, this chapter will look at the bureaucratic processes which reinforced English rule at provincial level. In the final section of this chapter, the governance of Irish asylums will be considered in relation to the wider question of Ireland's status as a colony or regional identity.

Homi Bhabha has cited rigid social administration in a colonial context as the outcome of colonial discourses aimed at presenting the colonised as degenerate in order to justify the imposition of colonial power (1994: 101). The imposition of an organised system of record-keeping and accountability suggests the presence of a rogue social element which needs to be recorded and held accountable. In the lunatic asylum, administrative processes were imposed from the outset, but the failings and problems associated with overcrowding among other problems – as discussed in the previous chapter – required the imposition of a more centralised administration by 1845. From the 1800s, administration and bureaucracy began with the process of admission and encompassed asylum maintenance, patient movement, patient experience, staff behaviour, and discharge. This section will build on De Cunzo's assertion of institutional admission as a ritual act (De Cunzo 2006), drawing on Goffman's discussion of mortification and cleansing practices (1976) and Van Gennep's 'rites of passage' (1960), in order to assess the extent to which the building's spatial layout supported admission practices.

Two venues for the effective running and administration of the asylum will be considered in detail: the administration block and the gate lodge. These spaces were key to patient admission, record-keeping, and management in the asylum. Architecturally, they are among the few individual elements of historic asylum buildings which have survived late twentieth-century mental hospital closure and redevelopment; for example, the administration block formed the central focus of redevelopment, as at the Wakefield Asylum and the Devon County Asylum (Franklin 2002b: 29–31). In the plans of purpose-built Georgian asylums, the administration block formed the central crux of a sprawling complex, radiating or extending out from the centre. This block was usually the most ornate and architecturally distinctive element of the asylum. Gate lodges, conversely, were generally unobtrusive, but as self-contained units – external to the asylum building itself – have survived as private residences in many former asylums. Archaeologically, administration blocks and gate lodges form large and tenable pieces of the built heritage.

The clerk, as an active agent in the asylum, is a liminal character in the historical record; on the one hand the producer of much of the physical record, and on the other relatively anonymous. The implements of his trade and their visibility and accessibility in museum, archival, and modern hospital contexts mean that the material remains of this job, in particular, make the clerk ironically one of the most visible figures in the material record. Indeed, the ledgers, account books, and documents produced by hospital clerks make up the most abundant material resources surviving from the early nineteenth-century asylums. Following this assessment of the material culture, both portable and architectural, the broader administration of the asylums within a national and civic context will be assessed.

Consultation of public account audits and reports to the Commissioners of Lunacy indicated a shift, around the mid-1840s, from handwritten accounts and ledgers to a standardised print form, whose format was evidently distributed to each asylum at this time. It is probable that this shift towards print formatting was standardised across other public institutions during the mid-nineteenth century. These standardised forms, the greatest volume of which were encountered in the accounts of provincial asylums, provided minimal information (extraneous to accounting figures) regarding the running of specific asylums. Their handwritten predecessors were generally detailed, providing accounts of life and problems encountered, with an additional report from the asylum managers. As such, the accounts taken into consideration here concerned the asylum's bureaucratic management prior to the introduction of this administrative reform.

The drive towards a more standardised form of public accounting arose from the consolidation of the new industrialised economy and a concern with organising the political economy in a more 'scientific' and rational manner (Alborn 2010: 70). This is reflected in texts on political economy from the period (Bigelow 2003: 119–22). Joyce has identified this drive towards the consolidation of the public record in the mid-nineteenth century as a supporting feature in the controlling objectives of the liberal European state (2003: 20). With regard to Ireland, the regulation of the administrative system indicated concerns over the resurrection of the Irish economy following the 1845–48 famine (Gray 2004: 153). Standardised printed accounts distributed to the asylums represent a primary material culture indicator of these processes. After the 1845 Act saw increased construction of lunatic asylums throughout the British Isles, asylum administration was affected significantly. The Act established the Commissioners for Lunacy, as an adjunct to the Home Secretary's overseeing of the new county asylums (Rutherford 2008: 15). This Act, and the proliferation of asylums afterwards, may have contributed to the adoption of a more efficient and standardised administration at the highest levels, so that the asylums could be audited in comparison with each other more effectively and in increased numbers.

A concern with efficiency in public administration occurred against the backdrop of a growing number of literate poor at this time (as discussed in Chapter 2). An increase in the level of literacy in this later period marks a shift from upper-middle class concern with public institutional provision to an atmosphere of accountability, where lay literacy ensured that public awareness through reading reports and texts may have influenced decisions. Public opinion and accountability enabled a wider outlook on asylums and was a concern in the British Parliament regarding lunatic asylum management as early as the inquiry into the York Asylum and the publication of a parliamentary report in 1815 (First Report 1815). Increased production and reduction of the cost in newspapers and the establishment of an increasing number of public libraries in large (and growing) cities, notably in the growing industrial north of England (Hewitt 2000: 66–7), further supports the assertion that the public were reading and interested in government activity. Awareness of their own accountability at this point heralded greater government conscientiousness in the maintenance of records and vigilance of inspections. The replacement of the Poor Law Commission with the parliament-represented Poor Law Board in 1847, following the exposure of abuses at the Andover Workhouse (Rees 2001: 61), reflects this greater awareness of government accountability for public institutions more broadly. The bulk of material culture surviving from lunatic asylums in the early decades of the nineteenth century is architectural and documentary. These sources will be employed in this chapter as bureaucratic material culture, as they represent the wealthiest source of portable material culture relating to the asylums from the early nineteenth century. Viewing the documentary record as a material source is an approach drawn from multidisciplinary research concerning the 'book' as a social and economic artefact (as discussed in the introductory chapter), as well as a textual source.

The administration block

The administration block was generally the most prominent element of asylum architecture. The administration block drew the eye of visitors and was a focal point for the architecture, as well as a first port of call. Aesthetically, this element of the asylum building represented the order of the institution, both in the regularity with which other buildings or wings proceeded from it, and in ornamental features like cupolas, pediments, or large windows. Generally, the administration block stood at the centre of each asylum plan and was the focal point of pathways or roads. The administration blocks were a common feature of other institutional buildings of the early nineteenth century, such as infirmaries and workhouses, and were thus familiar as an entry point for visitors or government officials. They generally stood to the front of the complex, drawing the eye and masking the utilities at the rear of the asylum. The administration block acted, variously, as an office space, a visitor's reception, an admission point, a meeting place, and sometimes as an accommodation block for the manager and his family. As such, the administration block was both separate from and intrinsic to the primary mission of the asylum, which was the management of the insane. The administration block was a liminal or threshold space between the outside world and the interior of the asylum. As a space for the bureaucratic management of the asylum by clerks who lived externally, as well as a space for the induction of patients and their display to family or visitors, the administration block acted as the boundary point between the patient and the outside world. Bureaucratic materials and spaces and admission processes will be examined in detail, followed by an exploration of the administration block as both a workplace and a domestic dwelling.

The administration block, as mentioned, usually occupied a central position in the asylum site, the main architectural feature to draw the eye both inside and outside the walls. Tall cupolas or pediments marked out this element of the building as the main point of focus, and thus entry. It was frequently the only element of the asylum building that was largely visible beyond the high walls of the asylum. Two examples illustrate the prominence of the administration block in asylum architecture. The Lincoln Asylum's administration block was dominated by a neo-classical pediment that could be seen from the south of the city, overlooking the steep Lincoln cliff. The asylum proper proceeded northwards from the administration block, invisible from the south. The Maryborough District Asylum, like other provincial asylums designed by Francis Johnston, was topped with a copper-domed cupola, with a clock on each of the cupola's four sides. The cupola was clearly visible over the asylum's high walls. East of the town of Maryborough, the asylum stood near a new reform prison and an infirmary and contributed to the growing institutional landscape of that part of the town. The visibility of the cupola above the administration block acted as both a beacon and a symbol of civic order.

Placing the administration block at the focus of the asylum was also a stylistic decision; positioning the entrance and primary government at the centre of the building was consistent with neo-classical design. In addition to style, the administration block was a feature shared by other public institutions. Workhouses built from the end of the eighteenth century and until the introduction of new Poor Laws in the 1830s and 1840s all evidence an emphasis on separation, starting with the central administration block, though the overwhelming majority of the inmates in these institutions were of the same pauper class (Morrison 1999: 30). This feature was carried over by asylum architects whose experience with public institutions was limited to prisons and workhouses or other neo-classical buildings like country houses. The stylistic resemblance between asylums and other buildings representing the establishment marked them out as part of the same framework of social order and civic improvement. What set asylums apart from workhouses, prisons, and even country houses were the principles of moral management written into the internal divisions within the buildings, as discussed in Chapter 2, and the designed landscapes which surrounded them. High walls and ha-has – reinforced ditches obscuring boundaries and utilities to provide an uninterrupted view from the main house (Curl and Wilson 2015) – were part of country-house architecture as well as asylum architecture, and reflect the importance of security from without, as well as within.

In the earliest radial plan asylums, such as the Glasgow Asylum and Cornwall County Asylum in Bodmin, the administration of the asylum was carried out in the central block from which the accommodation wings radiated. This had the effect of placing the administration and running of the asylum at a central space and at an equal distance from the corridors under observation. In theory, the idea behind this design was the importance of patient classification and the need to maintain centralised observation (Markus 1983: 205). These early asylum administration blocks had a few features distinguishing them from the outside as central governing spaces, but nothing on the scale of later asylums, as discussed below. The Richmond Lunatic Asylum (1816) in Dublin, for instance, had a crest of the Duke of Richmond, for whom the asylum was named, carved above the door, while the Nottinghamshire County Asylum (1812) had a sweeping staircase and carved doorway. As asylum architecture was trialled in the early nineteenth century, architects experimented with other building styles, such as the linear-plan with wings extending out from a central administration block, or Francis Johnston's K-shape, similar to a radial plan but with connecting corridors at the extremes of the extending wings (Figure 3.1). In each case, however, the administration block remained as the central focus. Increasingly, stylistic features like cupolas or weather vanes were employed to mark out the administration block. Unlike the observation-heavy central blocks of the radial-plans, the cupolas, towers, and weather vanes which topped administration blocks at asylums like Carlow District Asylum (1832), Maryborough District Asylum (1833), and other provincial Irish asylums designed by Johnston and his nephew Murray were not designed around observing from a centralised point (Figure 3.2). Rather, the cupolas and towers drew the eye from other parts of the asylum and from the outside. A symbol of authority and order, the administration block's cupolas, towers, and weather vanes acted as visual cues for the governance of the asylum.

Classification of patients according to sex was one of the central tenets of the reformed asylums and other major public institutions. Architecturally, the administration block acted as an effective physical buffer between the two sexes accommodated in the asylum. The separation of patients according to sex was deemed of primary importance in the treatment of the insane in some early instructional texts (Jacob 1833: 27; Tuke 1819: 2); many of the authors who penned instructions on asylums took the separation of male and female patients as a given

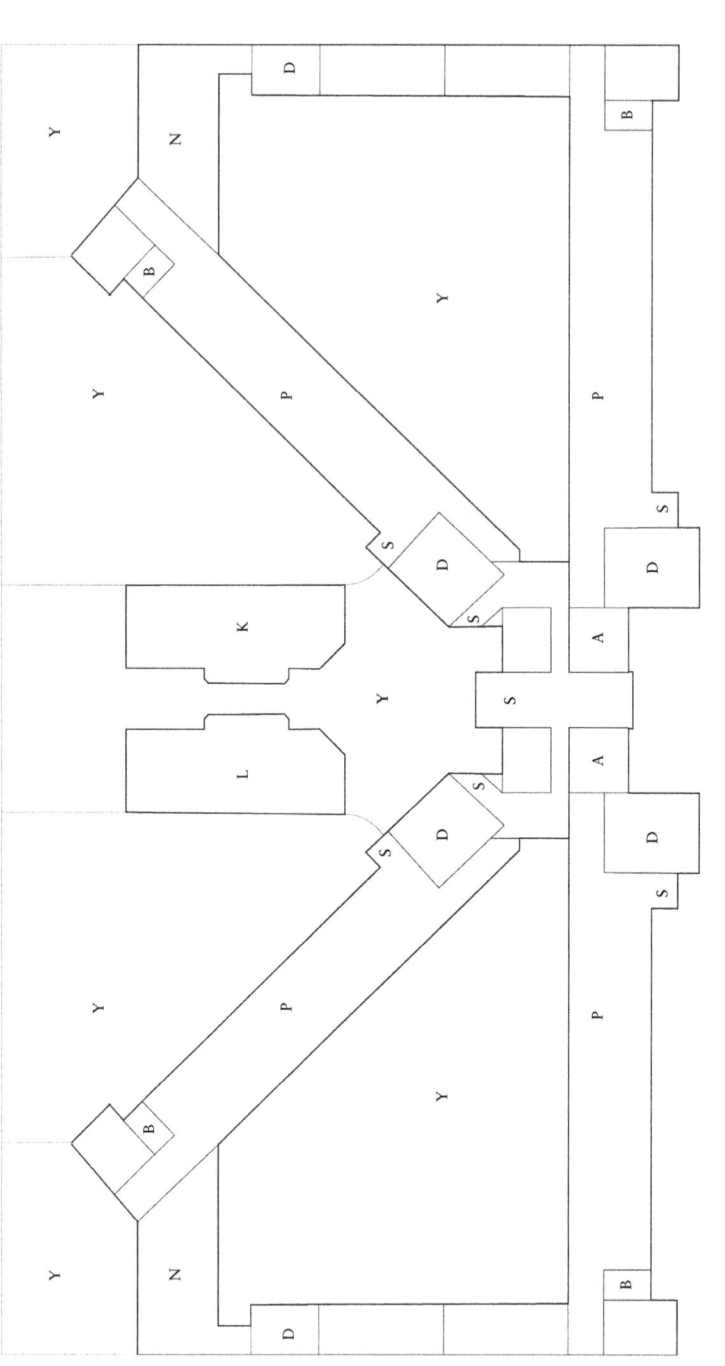

Figure 3.1 Carlow District Lunatic Asylum ground floor (1831). Administration (A), Baths (B), Day Rooms (D), Kitchen (K), Laundry (L), Noisy Patient Rooms (N), Patient Rooms (P), Stairs (S), Yard (Y).

Administration

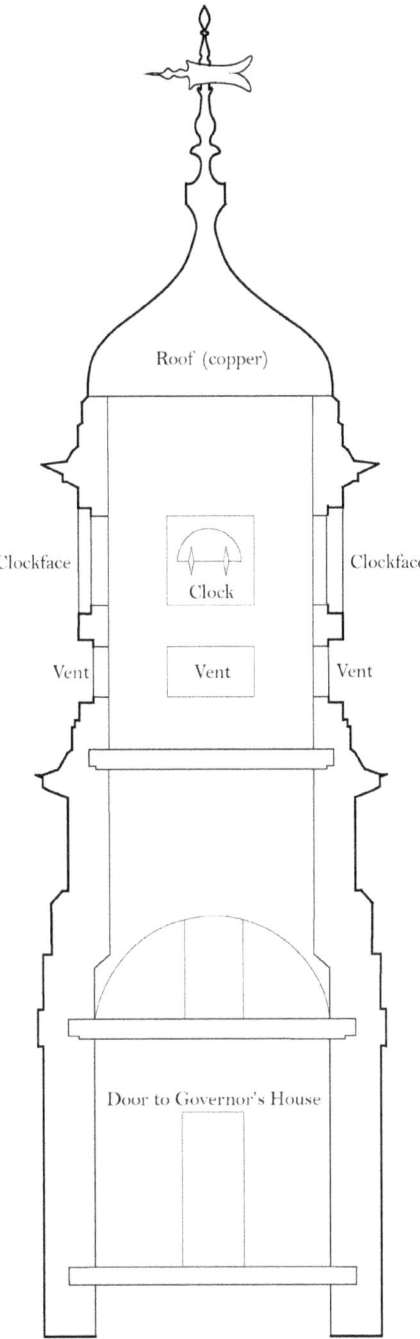

Figure 3.2 William Murray's schematic for a cupola at Maryborough District Lunatic Asylum (1832).

(Conolly 1847; Ellis 1838). As such, a feature like the administration block, creating a threshold space between the two sexes, was key to how asylums were designed. The separation of the sexes and the position of the administrative block as a buffer space became a singular tenet in symmetrical asylum design for the rest of the century. By the 1890s, after almost a century of reformed asylum design, the administration block retained its central focus and status as a liminal or buffer zone. Noted asylum architect and pioneer of later Victorian ideas about expanded asylums, G.T. Hine, designed his new asylum at Claybury so that the 'administrative department' was serviced by two separate corridors leading from the two separate departments, so that neither sex nor their staff need meet. Hine made a point of noting this, stating that the separation of the sexes was of central importance (1901: 167–8). In some spaces, such as the administration block, complete separation was not always possible, resulting in criticism.

The example of the actions of the Irish Board of General Control in 1817 demonstrates the weight attached to the administration block in the process of provincial asylum design in Ireland. In their assessment of suitable buildings for use as lunatic asylums from 1817, the Board rejected the reuse of the recently closed Roscommon Gaol, recommended to them by Undersecretary to the Lord Lieutenant of Ireland Robert Peel, as a suitable building for reuse as an asylum. The Board rejected the gaol on the recommendation of architect Johnston (National Archives of Ireland Commissioners for General Control: OPW 999/784, December 1817). In Johnston's plans for provincial asylums, submitted later that year, his sense of the ideal symmetry of an asylum was indicated by his addition of symmetrical accommodation for male and female patients, radiating out from the central administration block. The gaol at Roscommon was not considered suitable due to the lack of a proper means of classification, according to Johnston. Patients could not be accommodated 'with any degree of comfort or much prospect of relief, it would literally be a Hive of Angry bees [sic]' (National Archives of Ireland Commissioners for General Control: OPW 999/784, December 1817). The Roscommon Gaol building was small, designed in a T-shape, with offices to the front and cells facing each other as they extended in a single wing from the rear of the administration block. Johnston modified the plan, adding a number of new cells to the rear, separated from the original cells by a dividing wall and outside by a walled yard, presumably to allow for the accommodation of male and female patients. Internally, the administration block was not symmetrical. Johnston further queried that if the building were suitable for a lunatic asylum, why it was not kept in use as a gaol.

As an alternative to the use of existing buildings, Johnston proposed two different designs for provincial asylums: the X-shape for 150 patients and the K-shape for 100 patients (by far the most common design adopted). Johnston's designs allowed for separation of male and female inmates in separate wings, branching out from a central administration block. Johnston's influence in his preference for a symmetrical and linear-radiating building can be seen in his public works. His previous experience with lunatic asylums, repairs to George Semple and (later) Thomas Cooley's design for the private St Patrick's Asylum in Dublin (Boyd 2006: 90–1), reflected Johnston's influences. Asylum buildings were to be regimented in plan, symmetrical and extending from a central point, but necessarily separated internally to ensure security. Johnston's provincial asylum plans were an early example of an institutional building allowing for the complete separation of patients from the administration block (St Patrick's Hospital Archive Plan: F/9).

During the 1815 competition for the design of the Wakefield Asylum, the Visiting Magistrates rejected five designs in favour of the plan that finally won out, by architects Watson and Pritchett (West Yorkshire Archive Service West Riding: C85 1/1/1). The individual features of the prospective asylum designs will be discussed in more detail in the next chapter; they may also be considered with regard to how the architects engaged with the idea of a centralised administration block. The omission or positioning of the administration block was key to how the prospective asylum plans could be operated. One of the designs, by Hull-based architect Francis Hainton, was the only one of the five rejected designs not to place the administration block at the centre of focus, rather positioning the administration of the asylum at the rear and requiring the visitor to pass through the exercise yards of the asylum in order to reach the main door (West Yorkshire Archive Service Catalogue: QD1/694). All of the other designs placed the administration of the asylum primarily at the centre, with the patient rooms radiating from this block. London-based architect James Bevans submitted a radial plan (West Yorkshire Archive Service Catalogue: QD1/692), the only non-corridor plan of the remaining rejected designs. It is possible that considering the preference of the Visiting Magistrates for an H-design (as per the accepted design by Watson and Pritchett), was what won Bevans a second placing in the competition (West Yorkshire Archive Service West Riding: C85 1/1/1). His radial plan placed asylum administration at the very centre of the asylum building, with wings proceeding out in all directions from that point. The centrality of the administration block to the new asylum designs is evident in the ideas put forth for the Wakefield Asylum. Indeed, in the final built design, the small amount of internal space for the practice of administration in the central administration building (forming the bar of the H in the H-plan) was later criticised (Bolton 1928: 606).

From an architectural perspective, in line with the expansion of British and Irish towns and cities in the early nineteenth century, the administration block also fulfilled a stylistic role, forming the centrepiece of a symmetrical and aesthetically pleasing design. In the first decades of the nineteenth century, asylums were being designed against the backdrop of Georgian cityscapes, such as the redesigned Dublin City Centre focused around the extension of Sackville Mall to the River Liffey. The extension of Sackville Mall created a broad, wide European-style boulevard (Boyd 2006: 106–8), ideal for outdoor promenading and a staging area for increasingly more elaborate facades on public buildings like the General Post Office. The redevelopment of Dublin allowed for broader vistas and more open spaces. As well as filling an aesthetic role, the improvement of Dublin has been interpreted as both an effective means of population control (Kincaid 2006: xi–xxiii) and the continuity of an expression of imperial power (Kearns 2006: 179). This redevelopment occurred in the wake of the reconstruction of London after the 1666 Great Fire. Buildings in London and Dublin reflected the concept of order in their streetscapes, and designs such as the Custom House in Dublin (designed 1781) reflected this in their regimented arrangement. The Custom House consisted of wings radiating in symmetry from a central entrance point, designed as the focus of the building. The administration blocks for asylums provided this central focus for asylums from a stylistic point of view. Johnston, as a successor to James Gandon – the predominant Georgian architect in Dublin – may have perceived the lack of a central focus building at the Roscommon Gaol as stylistically outdated, unsuitable for a public building, as well as impractical for classification. The similarity between Johnston's institutional buildings and his public works, such as the General Post Office, has been noted in the regularity of form and imposing facades (Boyd 2006: 196). That this style of public building was fashionable can be seen in the popularity of the Wakefield Asylum designs in instructive texts on asylums, and the discussion of Bevans's and Stark's designs in parliament in the 1810s.

Whatever the motivation behind the central placement of the administration block, its position as the focus of movement into the asylum proper meant that it was a key venue in the admission of patients into the asylum. Following the initial physical admission of an individual to the asylum at the gate lodge (which will be discussed in detail in the following section), the administration block represented the site of official entrance or exit from the asylum as an institution for both the staff who worked in the block and the patients. Kitchen and laundry staff may have used the entrances to those parts of the building, but the administration block was still the focus of their management. The admission process, as a bureaucratic exercise expressed through form-filling and medical reporting, took place in the administration block, even if it is unclear if the admission block was the physical access point for the use of all classes of visitor or patient admissions. In the early asylum plans, these blocks took on a textbook plan, usually including an entrance hall, a waiting room, an office, and staff quarters. Common to most admission blocks were a waiting room, board or committee meeting rooms, the offices or living spaces of the manager (and sometimes his family), an inspection lobby, and a physician's room (based on Watson and Pritchett 1819; Irish Architectural Archive Murray Collection: 0092/046–0420–422; Copies of all Correspondence 1828: 234; Irish Architectural Archive Wilkinson Collection: 0085/138–116; St Patrick's Hospital Archive Plan: F/9). The administration block was the entrance route, the records centre, the bureaucratic centre, the inspection area, and the domestic dwelling of the manager and matron. There are variations to this. For example, the original plans for the Wakefield Asylum placed the manager and matron in separate quarters, in the towers of the asylum building, but with direct access to the administration and access corridors.

In relation to patient admission, the administration block represented a transitional zone through which an admission case must pass. This was the second point of transformation and transition, the first being the entrance gate which separated them physically from the outside world. The administration block was a site of admission whether the patient physically passed through it or not, as this was the venue for the processing of a patient and inducting them bureaucratically into the institution. This space represented the intervening period of *limen* or 'margin' in which the subject would transform from individual to inmate – in this case patient – through passage through an unfamiliar realm. Following transformation in this marginal space, a patient would be aggregated into the social world of the interior: the asylum (Turner 1969: 94–5). As a site of entrance, the rooms within the block allowed for overlap between the outside world and the asylum interior. Spaces of overlap or threshold were represented in waiting rooms and the office of the physician, who was not normally resident in the building but on whose inspection the continued confinement of the patient depended.

There is no indication in the plans or documentary evidence for asylums for a standard spatial procedure to be followed in asylum admission rituals in the early nineteenth century. In contemporaneous workhouses in England and Ireland, admission to a workhouse entailed the applicant to be present at the workhouse for inspection at a regular board meeting. Admission cases would be allowed through the front hall of the administration block and the applicant would proceed to a special wing, where they would be classified and their details recorded (O'Brien 1986: 114). The applicant would then be inspected by a medical officer, who would be most vigilant against any infectious disease (Stallard 1865: 9). Contagion spread quickly in public institutions, and during the cholera outbreaks of the 1830s and 1840s, applicants to workhouses and potential patients to public asylums were carefully screened and scrutinised. In the Wakefield Asylum, for example, there was a concentrated effort not to admit patients from districts affected with cholera in the year 1833 (Corsellis 1833: 3–5), likely due to a widely held opinion outside of the asylum that the institution was the source of the outbreak in the town, a claim that the manager Corsellis went to pains to debunk (1833: 3–5). In Ireland, the cholera outbreaks were carefully monitored centrally by the government. An outbreak of cholera in the town of Maryborough in 1832–33 would have been a serious concern for the manager of the asylum, which had just opened at that point (National Archives of Ireland Cholera Papers: 2/440/9).

The workhouse admission procedure culminated in a cleansing process. If admitted, the new inmate was bathed in the workhouse, clothed in workhouse clothing, and reallocated to the standard inmate rooms. This was a normal, standard procedure, subject to adaption and change. It is likely that a similar procedure was adopted for public lunatic asylums. The plans of public asylums and the built remains suggest that this was the case. The basement storey at the Maryborough Asylum contained twelve rooms, a bath, and access to either side of the asylum. The plan of the asylum states that the area was paved. Photographic survey of the basement of the former Maryborough Asylum (now St Fintan's Hospital, Portlaoise) confirms this. There were twelve small rooms marked on the plan as having small windows and thick framed doors; the presence of a bath and a lavatory at this level suggests the accommodation of patients here, though it is not recorded elsewhere (Irish Architectural Archive Murray Collection: 0092/046–0123). It is possible to suggest that on initial admission, applicants for the Maryborough Asylum, like workhouse applicants, were housed temporarily in a separate area (the basement) before bathing and inspection.

Applicants entering the workhouse in pre-famine Ireland, according to Gerard O'Brien, were admitted through the front hall of the administration block (1986: 114). It is unclear which entrance in the asylum was used, as an explicit accounting of the admission process to public asylums has not been located. There is no evidence to indicate that the patients were admitted through any other entrance, though the stately nature of the architecture indicates an active class distinction, despite the fact that these asylums were constructed for the admission of paupers. In Richmond, the notations by Johnston of the class types to be housed in the front and rear wards (wealthy to the front, pauper to the rear), may suggest a separation of applicant patients according to their social classification; there is an entrance to the rear of the asylum, and the presence of the baths in the rear laundry block supports the assertion that pauper applicants may have been separated. In the public asylums at Carlow and Maryborough, the administration block basement could be accessed through two exterior doorways, opening onto an outdoor terrace at ground-floor level and into a stairwell. The doorways were located to the left and right respectively of the day rooms flanking the administration block. It is possible that these doors were used for admission; however, the proximity of the baths, and the transgression of interior patient space that would be involved in the movement of the patient from the stairwell to the baths, cells, or inspection lobby, does not comply with the strict classification espoused by reformers such as Tuke. As there is no documentary evidence to support alternative access points for patients or pauper visitors, it is not possible to claim patient separation with any certainty.

The most certain material aspect of admission procedure was the filing of paperwork. This entailed the completion of details on a form by a relative or the patient, if lucid. Literacy rates (discussed in Chapter 2) suggest that the patients, and even their admitting relatives, may not have held the literacy level required to fill out the forms in the first half of the nineteenth century at least. Therefore, it can be assumed that in the case of illiterate patients, the form was written on their behalf by asylum staff or a member of the community who could vouch for them. Up to the 1840s, a magistrate, clergyman, or local medical attendant was required in any case to verify the insanity of the patient prior to their admission (Jacob 1833: 40; Levine-Clark 2004: 125). At Maryborough Asylum, the practice for admission required application for an admission form from the asylum, prior to any transfer (Abbott 1833b). Where the relative or patient could not complete a form, their supporting magistrate or clergyman would aid them in completing it.

It is not clear where exactly in the asylum the prospective patient was divested of the information recorded in admission documents. Admission information was written formally into admission books by a clerk in the office, so an interim form or record was likely kept. Admission books were printed to a formula and were usually large or cumbersome enough to suggest that they were probably not moved far from their place of permanent storage. The admission books for the Richmond Lunatic Asylum were printed to a standard before the asylum opened in 1815; they were large, measuring 0.55 m length and 0.45 m width closed. The Richmond Lunatic Asylum minute books totalled 0.88 m width on full opening, requiring a large work space for use, and ample storage space. It is probable that these were stored in the offices in the administration building, with other ledgers and account books, and moved only occasionally.

Asylums had many different ledgers, each to record a different aspect of asylum management. The number of ledgers held at the Armagh Asylum was detailed after the opening of the asylum in a letter from 1827. The ledgers at the Armagh Asylum included a general registry, a provision book, a want book, a store ledger, a delivery book, a proceedings book, a letter book, and a visitor's book (Copies of all Correspondence 1828; Williamson 1976: 117). Given the amount of cross-referencing that was required to maintain coherent records, it is probable that the books were not moved very far from each other, and that information was either filled in at the office or transcribed from another form. As with medieval illuminated manuscripts, the size and number of the books bound their location and use to a single specialised user group and administrative space (Greenia 2005: 735). A review of the plan of the Richmond Lunatic Asylum suggests that the most suitable space for housing the large ledgers, including admission books, was in the administration block, possibly in the forward rooms flanking the main asylum doorway. The close proximity of a board room and a visitor's room, where the manager and visiting members of the Board of General Control might review the day-to-day management and accounts of the asylum, shows the importance of good record-keeping in public institutions. As such, temporary forms which would then be input into the admission books were likely employed in admission practices. The procedure of maintaining a series of forms, which were later recorded in ledgers, was practised in psychiatric hospitals in Britain in the 1950s (Cross *et al.* 1957: 147). It is possible that this was an inherited practice.

The level of detail recorded in the Richmond Lunatic Asylum admission books reflects a diligent concern with record-keeping in the institution. The first patient, Andrew McKinley, was admitted in February 1814; he was initially admitted first to the House of Industry, and then to the asylum. His admission notes recorded that he was a soldier from Armagh, previously resident in the House of Industry, whose length of illness was unknown. This kind of detail was not uncommon. An early example of a patient form can be found in an affidavit drawn up by Dr John Jacob, physician to the Maryborough Asylum in 1833.

Affidavit.[sic]

County of
To wit. _____of_____
came before me this day and made oath on the
holy Evangelists, that to the best of know-

```
ledge and believe _____ of _____ in
the county of _____ parish of _____
barony of_____ nearest post town _____
has for some time past been in a state of insanity, and that the
said_____ is a pauper, and has no
friend who will or can be obliged to support      in a private
lunatic establishment, and that       has been a resident of the
said county of _____ for the last_____
and that      has not been an idiot.
Sworn before me at_____ this _____
day of _____ 18
_____ { Justice of the County
```
(after Jacob 1833: 46)

The affidavit would then be recorded and filed. On completion of the affidavit, patient admissions were to be supported by two statements: one by a member of the establishment, such as a magistrate or priest, and the other by the patient's next of kin; as well as an examination statement by the physician in charge (1833: 46–8). The volume of bureaucratic material involved in admitting patients by 1833 placed the figure of the clerk at the centre of the admission process, either as a scribe or as an office manager, maintaining and filing records so that they could be updated as required. This increased bureaucracy also meant that the process of admission was in itself a ritual which one must pass through in order to gain the next stage of institutionalisation.

As mentioned previously with regards to cholera, the hygiene of asylum admission and discharge cases was a primary concern to both the asylum and the government. Construction of asylums on well-drained land so as to prevent the cultivation of disease led to the erection of these buildings on high ground or near water sources; by 1845, the search for new sites for the asylums to be built on across England was focused around finding well-drained sites (Philo 2004: 584; Piddock 2007: 56). This was possibly a reaction to dysentery and cholera outbreaks in the 1830s. In seeking a site for the Wakefield Asylum, the Wakefield Magistrates decided on the site at Stanley, on a hill overlooking the town, due to its proximity to a water source and good drainage on high farmland (West Yorkshire Archives Service West Riding: C85 1/1/1). The importance of cleansing when inside the asylum was evident in the prolific provision of baths in the buildings; in his earliest plans for the provincial Irish asylums, Johnston provided up to ten baths for the patients' use (St Patrick's Hospital Archive Plan: F/9) – indicating his early awareness of the shortcomings of the Richmond Lunatic Asylum even just a year after its opening, which was only provided with four baths for the entire asylum located to the rear. The importance of washing as a treatment method in the late eighteenth century was seen by Foucault as almost baptismal and involved the use of baths and water as a treatment for the cleansing of madness from the body, with soap as a central component (Foucault 2006: 157–8).

Following the bureaucratic process of admission, a potential patient was assessed by a physician and submitted to cleansing processes, leading them through a second transitional (liminal) space, such as a bath or a dressing room, before their admittance into the final stage of admission and institutionalisation, which was installation in one of the patient rooms. In his assessment of institutionalisation, Goffman remarked that submission of outside identity through a cleansing activity and the surrendering of personal effects such as clothing was part of the process of making an inmate: depriving a person of the support of their social world (1976: 24) and initiating them into the support of the institution. The process of cleansing and re-dressing also played a role in securing the continued hygiene of the institution, a primary concern in the early asylums catering to the pauper insane and an ongoing problem as the asylums gradually became overcrowded. The sites of these rituals of precaution and hygiene involved movement through the building, through several different spaces, commonly housed in administration blocks.

The location of baths in asylums varied from site to site. At the Wakefield Asylum, the baths were located in an interconnected room between the administration corridors and the bedroom corridors, allowing for immediate spatial integration of patients into the asylum proper. The baths, located on the ground floor, were divided into 'hot' and 'cold', marking the cleansing process between the two sensory experiences. The baths were sunk into the floor and accessed by a set of stairs (details from Stephen Beaumont Museum of Mental Health Photographic Archive), allowing the patient to be immersed without needing to lie down, reducing the risk of drowning and facilitating staff assistance within the bath and above. By sinking the baths into the floor, the keeper at the Wakefield Asylum was able to maintain a supervisory gaze over the patient. This also placed the keeper within a position of control, so that the patient might be safely removed from the bath, if need be, with minimal risk of assault to the keeper. However, to a new patient, this may have been an intimidating experience, reinforcing a new hierarchy that placed the keeper in a position of power over the patient, and to which they were expected to adhere. The placement of the Wakefield Asylum baths served a secondary purpose as a public bathing space. The baths were originally designed to allow for public use (West Yorkshire Archives Service West Riding: C85 1/1/1, 2/11/1815), as a means of generating income, though it is not clear if the baths were ever opened to the public after the asylum was built. The doors to the baths opened into the administration block and the wards. Ventilation was provided by three windows set in the south facing wall, and the rooms were cooled by the placement of a cold bath in the room adjacent to the cell corridor.

The location of the baths at Johnston's asylums in Ireland, the provincial Irish asylums, and the Richmond Lunatic Asylum, are clearly marked on the plans. In the K-shaped provincial asylum plan, there was a bath room on the basement level, easily accessible from basement staircases in the inspection halls to either side of the administration block. On the upper levels, the baths were located to the extremities of the wings, so that a patient was moved through the corridor spaces before being bathed, fostering familiarity with the space. In the interest of hygiene and given the placement of baths at the end of corridors, the patient was probably not bathed in the ward baths on admission, but rather in the bath beneath the administration block, to reduce any contamination. Conversely, the baths for the Richmond Lunatic Asylum were located near the laundry block, to the rear of the building (Irish Architectural Archive Murray Collection: 0092/046–0420). This would allow for the passage of the patient through the central access corridor of the asylum, into the laundry block, without passage through the cell corridors. From this point, it may be surmised that the patient could be moved to any of the corridors without coming into contact with any other patients. The baths at the extremities of the asylum allowed for drainage or ventilation through external doorways in this area, and minimised any noise made, which would be amplified by the sealed interiors of the cell corridors if the baths were located there. The position of the baths at corridor extremes may have minimised the extent of steam and prevented excess damp permeating to the corridors.

Further admission procedures in the interest of maintaining hygiene may have been practised, as at other contemporaneous institutions such as female refuges, workhouses, and other institutions for domestic confinement. In public welfare institutions, inmates could expect to have their hair cut. In the Irish female refuges, a woman's hair was sometimes shorn as a symbol of her commitment to the moral mission of the institution, as a desexualising ritual as well as a hygienic measure. In Poor Law workhouses (after the 1830s), the institution had no authority to cut an inmate's hair, unless on the orders of a doctor. This may be due to the fact that in nineteenth-century England and Ireland, shorn hair on a woman was seen as the sign of an outcast (Luddy 2007: 60). Therefore, submission to scissors in workhouses may also be seen as an act of voluntary commitment to reform and chastity. A doctor in a workhouse might order a woman's hair to be cut, presumably in the interest of the health of the institution and as a ward against fleas. Similar precautions may have been practised in asylums; asylum physicians were often associated with workhouses and other charitable institutions where this practice was common. Dr Crowther, for instance, the visiting physician at the Wakefield Asylum, was the founder of several almshouses (Kirby 2008), while the physicians of the Richmond Lunatic Asylum also worked in the Dublin House of Industry (National Archives of Ireland: Richmond District Lunatic Asylum Minute Book 1). Therefore, it is probable that the practice of hair-cutting was carried out if required on the admission of patients where the physician saw fit.

The distribution of clothing was another aspect of the admission process, tied to the maintenance of a clean environment. On admission to the provincial asylum in Maryborough, a new patient was provided with asylum clothes (Williamson 1976: 116). In 1844, the Maryborough Asylum paid the Middlesex Asylum at Hanwell for the provision of clothing patterns so that Maryborough could make their own versions of the Hanwell-style patient clothing for their own patients, provided by local supplier William Roe (The National Archives of the United Kingdom Audits of Maryborough: AO 19/48/14). Interestingly, materials for keeper clothing and shoes were sourced from different suppliers to those for patients, suggesting a difference in quality and materials. Physician John Jacob's recommendation in 1833 that a patient be provided with a strong suit of clothes prior to their admission suggests that this practice was not strict when Jacob was writing his didactic treatise (1833: 46), but was imposed later on, at least by 1844. This suggests that regional provincial asylums in Ireland like the asylum at Maryborough were slow to impose policies outside of basic management, such as providing patients with clothes; but in a short few years after their opening, these asylums were making an active attempt to homogenise their practice in line with management practice in England.

In the interests of hygiene, new patient clothes were either distributed to patients by the asylum, or their own clothes thoroughly washed by the institution. That clothing held any significance to patients or staff beyond hygiene can be speculated. In her work on female patients in German asylums in the nineteenth century, Ann Goldberg equates the patient's clothes on admission with self and social identification, so that their loss becomes part of the institutionalising process (1998: 45), much as Goffman has suggested. Possession of her own pyjamas was described as a symbol of sanity and mental freedom by the Irish writer and ex-patient, Hanna Greally, in her autobiographical narrative of hospitalisation at St Loman's, Mullingar in the mid-twentieth century (Ward 2006: 72), *Bird's Nest Soup* (2009). When she is denied her own pyjamas, being ordered to wear 'what everyone else wears', Greally's protagonist becomes agitated (Greally 2009: 92). Clothing represented a facet of outside identity, but critical caution must be utilised in the attribution of clothing confiscation with significance beyond hygiene, due to a lack of direct historical accounts. The cleansing process, rather than the submission of clothes, may be considered to be the seminal rite of passage in the process of admitting the patient bodily into the asylum. The immersion of the patient into asylum life was furthered by other material culture which the patient was obliged to use in their everyday life in the asylum; for example, the use of cutlery.

Food-eating utensils were central to the daily life of the asylum. Forks, knives, and spoons, plates, and cups were used by everyone from patients to the manager. Given the large volume of material required on an everyday basis, it is not surprising that plates and cutlery are among the most prolific forms of portable material culture still extant. They are easily identified as belonging to asylums as many of these objects sported an asylum stamp. The Stephen Beaumont Museum of Mental Health in Wakefield houses a large number of plates and pieces of cutlery from the Wakefield Asylum and other West Riding asylums built later in the nineteenth century. Those items designated for patient use were made of tin to avoid shattering. This material has degraded badly and bears no trace of the original enamel which might once have borne an asylum stamp. Glazed earthenware ceramic is the only remaining evidence of the practice of stamping (besides cutlery); ceramic plates and cups were likely used by staff and well-behaved or convalescent patients. Patients were allowed the use of metal cutlery, albeit of a specific nature and probably not unsupervised. Cutlery was stamped, variously, with the initials of the hospital, an asylum crest, or the name of the institution.

Cutlery dating to the early nineteenth century is difficult to locate, due to replacement of utensils. As such, it is likely that the cutlery discussed in this study was only used at the very end of the period in question (the mid-nineteenth century) but indicates a continuity of provision of custom-made objects for daily use in the asylum. The cutlery used in public asylums as early as the 1860s was of a specific type. With few exceptions, the most prolific cutlery type to survive is solid-steel non-matching sets of knives, forks, and spoons. The fork and spoon handles were matching 'fiddle' patterns (so named for their violin-esque shape); the stem flares into a flat handle (on which the stamp appears) on one end, with a pronounced shoulder preceding the tines or bowl (Figure 3.3). Knives vary from flatware to bone-handled and are not usually stamped. A separate and distinct knife suggests that the set likely dates to before the 1880s, before the standardisation of matching sets (Dunning 2000: 43). Cutlery from the Stephen Beaumont Museum, from the Wakefield Asylum, are stamped, 'J. Lewis and Sons Sheffield', traceable to James Lewis, a cutlery manufacturer active in

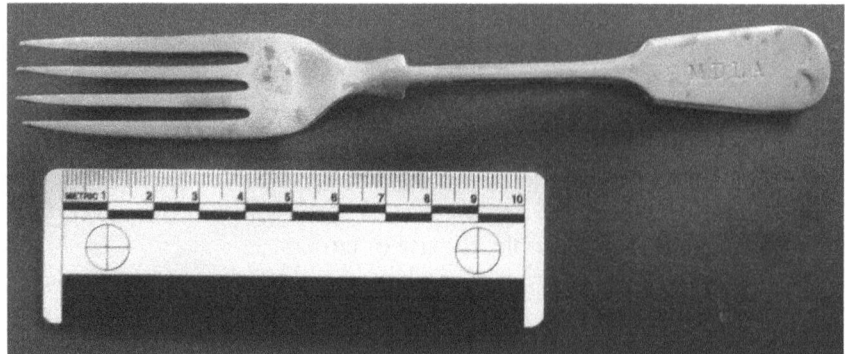

Figure 3.3 Example of fork from the Maryborough District Lunatic Asylum, with asylum stamp.

Sheffield in 1894–1909 (Busetto 2008) (Stephen Beaumont Museum of Mental Health). One example from Wakefield is ivory handled, possibly indicating a personal or status-use knife, made by Slack and Grinold of Sheffield, c. 1890 (Shackleford 2009: 95).

The use of status articles indicates stratified dining habits within the asylum. The distribution of cutlery was deliberate and carefully managed; the steel-handle knives from the Wakefield Asylum are numbered so that their use could be monitored. This practice may have had two motivating factors. Staff behaviour may have been a consideration; numbering of cutlery could prevent theft from the hospital. Patient safety in the use of these instruments was a major factor in the distribution of steel utensils. A later selection of cutlery for patient use from the Richmond Lunatic Asylum (dated to the 1920s, makers mark Daniel and Arter, Birmingham) (Busetto 2008) was modified so that the tines of the fork were filled in, up to within a few millimetres of the tip, so that the implement was useful for scooping and gripping, but not for stabbing. A knife from the same collection had a similarly modified blade edge, which was dull but for a short few centimetres in the middle of the blade. This precaution prevented the use of the blade as anything other than a tool for cutting very small measures, minimising the risk the patient posed to themselves or others in the event of their getting hold of a knife or fork they were not entitled to use.

Patients became actively initiated into asylum life through the use of materials like cutlery and food receptacles, which in turn minimised their scope for individual expression. Some personal effects have emerged in the material record, however, which suggest that items were also brought in from outside. Domestic items such as ceramic pipes appear in the archaeological record, which attest to the personal identities maintained by the inmates (staff and patients) in the institution. The bowl and a stem fragment of a clay pipe were unearthed during the demolition and development of the Wakefield Asylum and relocated to the Stephen Beaumont Museum. The fragment comprised a plain bowl with a spur and an incised design spelling the word 'Dublin' in an oval. This pipe may be one of hundreds cast by a pipe maker from Leeds in the mid-to-late nineteenth century, who was noted for taking advantage of the growing market of Irish migrant workers in the north of England (Weldrake 2012: 1). Similar pipes were found in an excavation in Sheffield's Riverside Exchange. An 'Irish style bowl' with a similarly incised rim and the word Dublin stamped in an oval was found and dated from the mid-nineteenth century (1840) to the start of the twentieth century (White 2015: 29). The probability of this pipe actually originating in Dublin is slim, owing to the geographical distance between the two places and the number of pipe manufacturers between Wakefield and Dublin. The provenance of a clay pipe is not always obvious owing to the proliferation of the industry from the eighteenth century across Europe and the Americas. Therefore, it is most likely that this pipe's provenance was a canny Leeds pipe manufacturer aware of a growing Irish market. The use of this pipe to the point of discard suggests that the user could have been Irish or had links to Ireland and, as such, took steps to assert his distinctive identity by using a pipe marked 'Dublin'.

Mass migration from Ireland in the mid-to-late nineteenth century as a result of famine, economic instability, and rural evictions brought many Irish people to the industrial centres of England and the United States. Historian of medicine Catharine Coleborne has described the impact of migration and displacement as causing homesickness and nostalgia in the colonial mindset of settlers in nineteenth-century Australia and New Zealand (2010: 44–7). The material legacy of mass migration from rural Ireland to cities like New York is further evidenced in domestic assemblages from the period (Orser 2007: 79–82). The Wakefield 'Dublin' pipe suggests that at least one individual at the Wakefield Asylum maintained an emotional attachment to Ireland, articulated through their purchase of an engraved pipe. One pipe is not enough evidence to suggest that the Irish population in industrial England suffered psychologically in their displacement, but it does suggest that the Irish diaspora were actively maintaining emotional ties to Ireland in their consumption habits. Furthermore, material such as the Wakefield pipe indicates the maintenance of a somewhat comfortable lifestyle for the patients and staff, rather than an austere institutionalising process scouring them of their individuality. This is also articulated in the architecture of the asylum, and particularly the administration block

At the Maryborough Asylum, the residence of the manager was

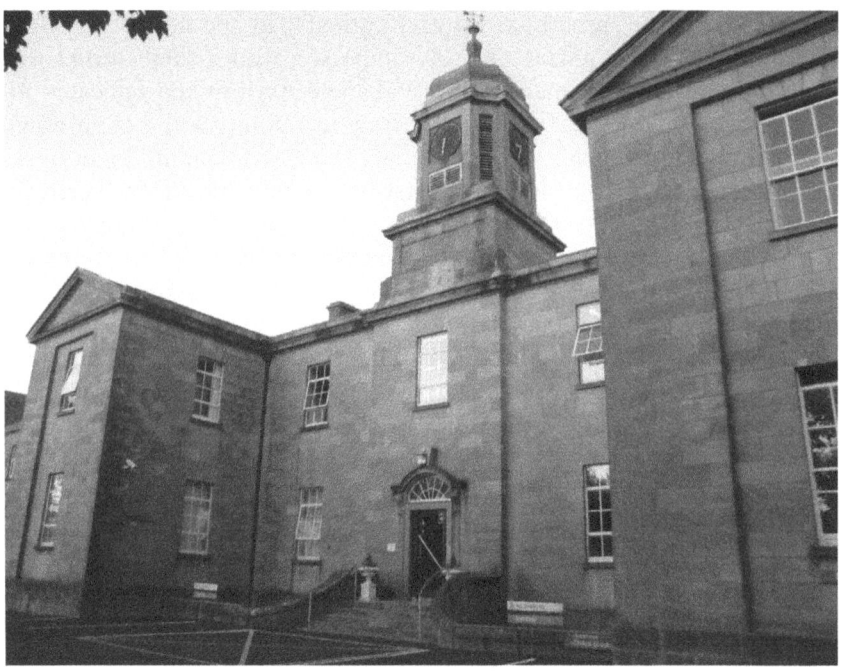

Figure 3.4 Facade of administration block at St Fintan's Hospital, Portlaoise, formerly the Maryborough District Lunatic Asylum.

modelled on period domestic architecture: the block emulates Georgian houses similar to the townhouses of late eighteenth-century and early nineteenth-century Dublin. These houses were divided into separate spheres: utility (basement), reception (ground), and living space for family and servants (upper floors). The administration block at the Maryborough Asylum (Figure 3.4), and other provincial Irish asylums built along Johnston's guidelines as enacted by his nephew William Murray, was divided upon similar lines. The basement was an institutional space for admission and cleansing, reception and offices were located on the ground floor, while personal offices for the master and matron, as well as living apartments, were located on the upper floors. As a building, it was similar in form and style to the adjacent Maryborough Infirmary (1808), which was also built along the lines of an upper-class domestic abode. The Infirmary was designed by another Irish architect, David Henry, who was himself proficient in public works and applied (unsuccessfully) to succeed Johnston as Public Works architect (National Archives of Ireland Chief Secretary's Office: CSO/RP/1825/1824). In architectural style, the asylum administration block was similar in aspect, if not in internal division, to Johnston's Townley Hall, a stately home in Co. Louth. Interestingly, neither the Maryborough Infirmary nor Townley Hall incorporates the diminishing window size typical of contemporaneous Dublin townhouse architecture, which is used at the Maryborough Asylum, the Carlow Asylum, and at other provincial Irish asylums.

The entrance to the Maryborough Asylum, through a large door set into a moulded frame topped with a semi-circular window, was echoed on the inside of the entrance hall by the doorway to the residence, which led to an ornate central staircase. The residences of asylum managers were strategically placed so as to allow for maximum accessibility to all corners of the building. At the provincial Irish asylums, the manager was privy to exclusive access downstairs via the central staircase and through side staircases, which led to an inspection lobby on either side of the block; the central staircase led to the front hall but was a more observable entrance. At the Wakefield Asylum, the quarters of the manager and matron were situated facing the administration corridors at the centre and abutting the spiral access stairways connecting the floors. The proximity of their domestic and official quarters to the access staircases was deliberate. The manager and matron's offices were designed with the active supervision of other staff in mind, as per the recommendations of Samuel Tuke to prospective architects (1819). The spiral staircases terminated in a basement corridor, crossing beneath the administration corridors and connecting the male and female parts of the hospital by an unseen access route.

By connecting the manager's domestic space with the institutional space of the asylum, the domestic character of the reformed asylum was reinforced, imposing domestic standards of maintenance on the building and grounds, in theory at least. It may be noted that the access privileges afforded support staff such as laundresses in the execution of their duties would have provided them access through these spaces, and to staircases such as the ones to the side of the manager's residence at the Maryborough Asylum. The position of the latter and their access routes to the fringes of the manager's house, as well as into the basement, bear a resemblance to contemporaneous 'servant's stairs' in domestic contexts in the late eighteenth century (Lucas 1999: 126). The backstairs may have served the dual purpose of a service route and a means of quick, easy access for the manager. Andrew Scull has suggested that the push towards domesticity in the early asylums was driven by an endeavour to gentrify madness as a condition common to all classes, but especially the upper classes (1989: 74–5). That it was widely known that the King was afflicted with his own debilitating condition by the early nineteenth century reinforces the point that sympathetic, humane, and proto-domestic treatment was essential in housing the mentally ill

(Macalpine and Hunter 1991: 329). The domestic life of the manager or governor of the asylum was built in to the architecture and decor of the administration block interiors and reinforces the point that domesticity as a feature was primary in the design process.

The administration block was a domestic dwelling, a space for admissions, a waiting area, and a meeting place; it was also an office space and workplace for the non-residing members of staff. The asylum clerks worked in the asylum and were essential to its running, but they did not live there. Anderson, in his work on Victorian clerks, notes the relationship between the employer and the clerk as paternalistic in nature and interdependent: the nineteenth-century clerk was indispensable to their employer, who repaid him with security, status, and social mobility (Anderson 1976: 31). Social mobility was of key importance to a young lower middle-class clerk. The asylum clerks occupied a position both between and parallel to the relationship between the general staff and the management. The clerk was literate, and a base level of education was required for them to take up the positon. In the material record of public institutions, clerks are the most visible characters, though their individual agency with regard to the material they transcribed was limited. The clerks, as transcribers and authors of the textual sources, were associated with and responsible for the maintenance of the ledgers and official minute books.

By far the most prolific material culture resource for asylum study (apart from the standing buildings themselves, where they survive) is the large volume of written records contained in ledgers, accounts, and letters, the extant bulk of which is now housed in local and national archive offices. Despite the volume of material, however, the men who composed much of this written record are largely invisible. Unless a document was explicitly signed by a named individual, most of these records were set down by clerks employed by those who authored or commissioned the written records. The identity of individual clerks can be found in their expression or 'hand' (Augst 2003: 8). Handwriting is the only vehicle for identifying individual clerks. Consistent use of a single handwriting style indicates a single dedicated clerk, while multiple different handwriting styles indicate a staff of clerks. For example, multiple changes in handwriting in the minutes of the Board of General Control for Irish Asylums suggests the use of the book by multiple clerks and administrators, indicating a staff of clerks working where the book was stored, rather than an individual character. The materials of office for a clerk are innocuous and are thus overlooked in the material record of lunatic asylums. The office supplies of a clerk in a lunatic asylum are not very different from those of an accounting firm. Paper was sourced from local or noted sources, sometimes from official suppliers to the government and other times from local bookbinders. The Wakefield Asylum ledgers were made by a local bookbinder and ledger maker (West Yorkshire Archives Service West Riding C85 1/1/2), while the Maryborough Asylum accounts were written in a ledger made by a printer based in London, John Smith of 49 Long Acre, a self-described supplier to the Stationery Office (The National Archives of the United Kingdom Commissioners for Auditing: AO 2/68). As artefacts attesting to the day-to-day work of these men, the ledgers provide impersonal accounts and a detached writing style.

Official stamps and insignia are among the few diagnostic features of individual asylum office practice. These stamps bore the asylum name and attested to the official seal of the office. An example from the Maryborough Asylum was made of brass and measured 0.09 m on the base. The size and weight of the stamp suggests that it was used for ink stamping, rather than use in wax. A wax seal from the Richmond Lunatic Asylum was 3 cm, made with a letter stamp to affix a green ribbon around the accounts of the asylum for 1845 (The National Archives of the United Kingdom Audits of Richmond: AO 19/48/17). The example from the Richmond Asylum is the only surviving example of the use of a wax seal in that asylum, while ink stamps on audits and letters evidence the use of an ink stamp. The volume of cross-referenced historical material surviving from asylums – in ledgers, accounts, and letters – suggests that the official paperwork relating to the management and administration of the asylum was housed in ready, accessible locations, for the convenient use of the clerks and administrators involved in record-keeping.

The clerk also represented a contact between the lunatic asylum interior and the outside world. The Clerk of the Peace responsible to the Wakefield Magistrates during the planning and construction of the asylum at Wakefield was the primary contact for architects and tradesmen inquiring about the asylum. This clerk, John Foljambe, advertised in the local papers and acted as intermediary between the Magistrates and the men working for them (for an example of his work, see Foljambe 1814; this is the request for proposals distributed to local papers). The clerk, while intimately involved in the running and management of the asylum, was also a liminal figure. Clerks recording information in the asylum minute books and the general staff responsible for attending to the needs of patients (the keepers and nurses) occupied separate spheres within the asylum, both socially and spatially. Through their direct engagement with management and their position of responsibility over the official records of the institution, the position of the administrative clerk in the asylum was spatially and hierarchically above that of the general staff, and above (if detached from) patients. The clerks communicated their superior position in the asylum hierarchy through the maintenance of records and the reporting of disobedience.

As an 'officer of trust', as physician John Jacob described them, the clerk was expected to report any breach of discipline among the general and support staff to the manager (1833: 58). This expectation of sub-superintendence (whether acted upon or not) would have placed the clerk outside of general staff networks, in a similar position to that of the gatekeeper, which will be described in more detail later in this chapter. Though not a member of management, the clerks were marginal figures in the running of the asylum due to their position 'above' the keepers and attendants. Their spatial location, close to the front doors and apart from the rest of the asylum, set them apart too. In addition, class was another divisive factor. Clerks were, by necessity of their position, literate. By the late nineteenth century, there is evidence to suggest that while a significant percentage (56 percent) of clerks working in England were from working-class backgrounds, the nature of their profession set them firmly within a class bracket more associated with the management, rather than the support staff, if not the general staff (Vincent 1993: 132). An increase in primary schooling and the greater availability of positions in consequence of the Industrial Revolution effectively resulted in the proliferation of a professional clerical class in British and Irish cities. In Ireland, too, the Lord Lieutenant also reserved the right to appoint a clerk if he so wished, creating an extra social and political dimension to the clerk's position (Grimsley-Smith 2011: 51). In the early-to-mid nineteenth century, when the number of provincial and public asylums was increasing, literacy levels were not so significant, suggesting that those who had attended school and were proficient enough to become clerks were from the lower middle classes, at least for the first half of the century. The position was a firmly middle-class pursuit in the United States in the same period (Augst 2003: 208–9) and may be considered an engine for social mobility from the middle of the nineteenth century onwards on both sides of the Atlantic.

Aesthetically, the administration block represents the physical look of the lunatic asylum. When asylum architecture was still experimental – when Francis Johnston was playing with ideas for how Irish provincial asylums could look, and Watson and Pritchett were competing with other architects for the contract to design the West Riding Asylum in Wakefield – the administration block was presented as a focal point for the running and management of the institution. From the outset, the administration block was to host a number of different but complementary activities, with each of them necessarily set apart from the day-to-day management of the patients. The admission of prospective patients through the administration block, whether physically or bureaucratically, was carried out in dedicated spaces set apart from the asylum proper. The administration block acted as a liminal, threshold space in the initiation of new inmates to the institution. The admission process was more nuanced than suggested by Erving Goffman's descriptions of institutionalisation, however, and was geared towards the effective physical management of patients for the health, safety, and comfort of themselves and others. The activities necessitated in the management and cleansing process, however, could also be read from the perspective of a prospective patient, for whom the loss of identity was a material reality. The final part of the admission process involved the incorporation of the patient into the bureaucratic records of the asylum, a different, less physical, but no less dehumanising process. The bureaucratic admission of a patient into the asylum was carried out by a clerk, a member of staff who was spatially and socially separate from the patient, who may never have met the patient, but on whose work the historical legacy of the patient's admission into the asylum depended.

Gates and offices

The following section will look at another marginal figure, the gate lodge keeper, whose physical presence and necessary position in the asylum has resulted in a prolific material legacy, but who remains a largely anonymous figure in most asylum histories. The gate lodge and its denizen, the gatekeeper, oversaw the first point of entry to the asylum. Lodges were situated at main gates; as asylums grew over the course of the nineteenth century, other lodges were also constructed at entrances further away. They were a common, if not universal, feature flanking the entrance to the grounds of public asylums; it was not standard practice to incorporate them stylistically into the design of the asylum until later in the nineteenth century. The gate lodges, as distinct, separate features represented an architectural commonality between asylums and country houses, further reinforcing the intentions of the architects and reformers to build a domestic institution. By the beginning of the 1840s, gate lodges were a standard feature of asylum complexes, as detached houses or built into the side of an entrance gate. The architecture of gate lodges and their inclusion in the plans of the asylums indicates several architectural influences, including the estate architecture of country houses as well as institutions like workhouses. This section will consider how the adoption of gate lodges as a feature of asylum building related to an increasing concern with making the architecture of the asylum domestic, and their role as entrance spaces and passage points in the admission process. Gate lodges, like admission blocks, were liminal zones, occupied by peripheral figures in control of passage both in and out of the asylum.

Apart from marking the entranceway to the asylum, the gate lodges were also the private abodes of the gatekeeper. The position was full-time, and the asylum provided for some of the needs of the gatekeeper, such as outdoor clothing. As such, the gate lodge was as much a domestic space as an institutional one. As private residences, the interior of asylum gate lodges was designed to accommodate one person (or a couple), with a bedroom and a kitchen. By the early nineteenth century, a long tradition of domestic labourer dwellings and gate lodges had settled to a uniform standard. The gate lodges of British country houses by 1800 generally reflected the architectural style of the main house, following several centuries of experimentation and ostentation (Mowl 1984: 474). Similarly, gate lodges in asylums became increasingly formalised through the first half of the nineteenth century, so that by the 1850s the inclusion of a gate lodge on the asylum estate was standard practice.

Gate lodges as an architectural feature are not commonly included in overviews of country-house architecture, which focus on the main houses themselves (see Christie 2000; Franklin 1981; Girouard 1978) and are mentioned only occasionally in cases of extraordinary architecture (for example, see the description of Townley Hall in Casey and Rowan 1993: 506; Craig 1982: 319). Guides from the eighteenth and nineteenth century suggest that gate lodges were important as the most accessible public face of the house. In the *Country Gentleman's Architect* of 1787, the author, Miller, listed six different porter's lodges of his own design, to precede country houses. These lodges all flanked gateways and consisted of two discrete structures to either side (1878). In a later work of the same type, published twenty-three years after Miller's compilation, another architect, Middleton, presented a similar collection of gate lodges alongside newer designs for a separate collection of Romanesque style 'Keeper's Houses' (1810) for country estate staff. There was a gradual separation of gate lodges from the structure of the gate itself as they developed as separate domestic dwellings; presumably, the ability to maintain a full-time gatekeeper was a subtle means of indicating wealth. By 1846, an encyclopaedia for the architecture of cottages and villas at country houses included a standardised design for gate lodges. Gate lodge architecture, much like asylum architecture, was formalised in the mid-nineteenth century; models for gate lodges illustrated the different specifications to be included in lodges, including a living room, bedroom, kitchen, storage space, and a privy. Gate lodge architecture became refined as a speciality, with architects such as the amateur Sir George Hodson in Ireland specifically designing gate lodges for houses and institutions. The outward appearance of country-house gate lodges, when they became commonplace, was intended to express an outward appearance of 'simplicity and elegance' (Louden 1846). In the gate lodges of the provincial Irish asylums, constructed to a uniform style by the 1830s, the style of the asylum was aped in the outward appearance of the lodge, down to the building stone used. The provincial Irish asylum gate lodges, as architectural features, also exemplified the features of the country-house lodge model, indicating a common architectural genesis. Given Johnston's previous experience with large country houses in Ireland, this is not surprising.

Asylum architecture, as has already been explored, was also heavily influenced by the contemporaneous institutional architecture of the period, such as workhouses and infirmaries. Asylum architecture in the early nineteenth century was aesthetically similar to workhouses built in the late eighteenth and early nineteenth century (Morrison 1999: 24–5). The Richmond Lunatic Asylum, given its close links with the adjacent House of Industry, bore a strong resemblance to the workhouse and to another on the south side of the city, both of which were purpose built in the eighteenth century (O'Brien 1986: 1; Robins 1986: 7–15; Walsh 2001: 7–8). As such, asylums like the Richmond Lunatic Asylum, that is purpose-built urban institutions with very close geographical and managerial ties to other institutions, must be considered as part of a complex. The installation of a gate lodge at the Richmond Lunatic Asylum, and the addition of a larger, purpose-built lodge in the middle of the nineteenth century, marked the asylum out as distinctive. The gate lodge, as a feature of country-house architecture, set the asylum apart as a different type of institution from others in the city.

The separate lodge in the grounds of the Richmond Lunatic Asylum does not appear on any of the early plans for the asylum prior to 1855 (Irish Architectural Archive Murray Collection: 0092/046–0411–20; Copies of all Correspondence 1828). A simple bungalow lodge of a similar style to the provincial asylums was designed in 1855 (Irish Architectural Archive Holybrooke Collection: 87/55–4461). A small lodge attached to the west side of the House of Industry, outside of the walls of the asylum (Irish Architectural Archive Murray Collection: 0092/046–0416), was the closest comparison with the later Johnston and Murray plan gate lodges constructed at the provincial asylums. A separate gate lodge for a live-in lodge keeper may not have been considered necessary until the asylum began to expand, as access and egress to the Richmond Lunatic Asylum was catered for by a common gate lodge at the bottom of Morning Star Avenue. The gate and lodge are clearly marked on the First Edition Ordnance Survey map of the area (1837). This lodge likely predates the construction of the Lunatic Asylum and acted as the primary point of monitored access to the House of Industry and other institutions on the avenue. Morning Star Avenue may have been a private avenue, in any case. The 1837 Ordnance Survey maps, used by Rev. M'Cready in his compilation of Dublin street names in 1892, does not label Morning Star Avenue, and it is not mentioned in M'Cready's exhaustive index (1987: xv, 70). Morning Star Avenue was probably originally a private avenue for the use of the institutions which lined it. A second line of controlled access was added for the asylum, as a budgetary consideration in the 1819 Richmond Asylum minute book indicates the asylum was, at that point, in control of its own access and egress (National Archives of Ireland: Richmond District Lunatic Asylum Minute Book 1). Internal division of the institutions on the avenue would have been necessary for the maintenance of security, as well as classification of inmate types. The single lodge, large enough for a domestic dwelling, became increasingly popular in institutional contexts. A description of Dublin's Richmond Bridewell, on the site of the Dublin Union workhouse on the south side of the river, notes a gate and a small discrete porter's lodge (Walsh 2001: 10). This suggests that Irish institutions were opting for a single lodge, in place of the previously fashionable flanking porter's lodges, as indicated by floor surfaces uncovered on either side of the old gates of the South Dublin Union Workhouse (Walsh 2001: 44).

English asylums were less uniform, and as such widespread change was slow. Some asylums incorporated both styles, and a second checkpoint for entry into the asylum was not an uncommon feature. The Wakefield Asylum (1819) had a gate lodge opening onto the Stanley Road, which ran alongside the asylum to the east, and a porter's lodge to the east of the main gate into the north asylum yard, overseeing a weighbridge. With the weighing machine on one side of the gate and the porter's lodge on the other, the gate from the wider asylum grounds into the yard was well supervised. The architects, Watson and Pritchett, were also responsible for constructing private homes, notably lodges for Rise Hall in the East Riding of Yorkshire. The gateway of Rise Hall was flanked by two neo-classical lodges, neither of substantial size or capacity (Thomas 2009). The porter's lodges at the Wakefield Asylum reflect this influence, as well as the influence of other institutional types. In-gate lodges were used in religious style complexes constructed at this time, such as at colleges in Oxford and Cambridge. In the seventeenth-century buildings of Oriel and Wadham Colleges, Oxford, the porter's lodge was a central feature in the new construction. The porter was situated so as to allow easy surveillance of access and egress. This was a new feature, less common in the older colleges (Durning 2009: 91). These monastic-style colleges were subject to the influence of other institutions, which also may have influenced the choice of porter's lodge style applied by Watson and Pritchett at the Wakefield Asylum.

As the first point of admission or exit from the asylum, the gate lodge occupied a significant position in the processes of patient admission and the surveillance of staff and visitors. In *Prisons, Asylums, and the Public: Institutional Visiting in the Nineteenth Century*, historian Janet Miron ties public interest in landscape and architecture with a broader nineteenth-century preoccupation with visual culture and 'visiting' in local areas, on both sides of the Atlantic (2011: 119–22). She notes that visitors to American and Canadian asylums in the nineteenth century were concerned with the architecture and grounds of public asylums, as well as with the interior and the patients (2011: 87). The addition of a gate lodge to asylum grounds, with the associations those buildings had with country-house architecture, lent a level of gravitas and decorum to the asylum landscape, for visitor's eyes only. Van Gennep's description of a liminal space, as a space between the sacred and profane which was necessary for the cleansing or preparation of a subject (1960: 1), may be applied to the entrance space of the asylum, overseen by the gate lodge. This was the first phase of the admission 'ritual', in which the prospective patient would separate themselves from the outside world, physically crossing the gate threshold (Turner 1969: 94). The three stages involved in the rites of passage here are employed as Van Gennep and Turner describe: separation [of the patient from the outside world], liminality [of state before admission], and re-assimilation [institutionalisation]. The re-assimilation stage, which in Turner's ritual process refers to the re-assimilation of an individual with their *communitas* (1969: 94), can refer in this context to a patient's or even a staff member's integration into the institutional *communitas* of the asylum, as per Goffman's descriptions of institutional assimilation (1961: 24; 50–1). In readings of Van Gennep, the ritual concepts involved in the rites of passage have been applied to mythology and texts, identifying characters such as Charon the boatman of the Ancient Greek underworld as figures of liminality, providing guidance to the journeyman in unfamiliar, transitional spaces (Saeedi 2009: 6). The asylum gatekeeper can similarly be viewed as an agent of liminality, being the overseer of the separation of patients from the outside world, and the literal gatekeeper in the process of community re-assimilation practised by staff members who enter and leave the asylum on a frequent basis.

The gate lodge of the Maryborough Asylum is a good example of the provincial Irish asylum gate lodges. This lodge was constructed next to the north-facing gate of the asylum, opening on to the Dublin Road, the main northeast road leading out of Maryborough towards Dublin, and facing Maryborough's convict prison (1832). Just west of the asylum gate was the gate for the County Infirmary. This small area to the north-east of the town of Maryborough was populated primarily by institutions and their associated architecture. This was not uncommon among the provincial asylums, which were constructed on the outskirts of major towns or cities, though many were gradually overtaken by residential and other institutional development. The Maryborough Asylum lodge was constructed of the same limestone as the asylum itself, lain in ashlar style, and was part of the initial overall construction phase of the original asylum (Figure 3.5). The architectural similarities between the two reinforced the role of the lodge as an outpost of the main asylum itself. The gate lodge acted as the initial initiation stage, through which the subject must pass. The plans of the Maryborough lodge depict elevations of the front (outside) view of the gate, illustrating the point that any view over the gate or wall was impossible. Only the eaves and roof of the lodge were visible over the wall (National Archives of Ireland Plans of Clonmel Asylum: OPW 5HC/4/884; Irish Architectural Archive Murray Collection: 0092/046–0134; Irish Architectural Archive Wilkinson Collection: 0085/138–4634). As such, before even entering the asylum grounds, the first call point for a patient or visitor was already visible in the low roof of the lodge. Maryborough Asylum physician John Jacob indicated that prospective patients were held at the gate by the gatekeeper, to await advice from the manager on their admission to the asylum (1833: 59). This practice gave management time to review any paperwork (the aforementioned affidavit, for example) before the admission process could be instigated. Such a practice also necessitated the maintenance of a clean lodge and the addition of a parlour to the structure, which was at once both a holding area for the institution and the domestic dwelling for the gatekeeper.

Allusions to the gatekeeper in the documentary record of asylums are not prolific. At the Maryborough Asylum, the provision of a private residence for the keeper (albeit a small one) marked the gatekeeper out as an asylum resident, much like the manager and matron. This separated the gatekeeper from clerks, and from other general staff who were resident outside the grounds, encompassing him in the inner asylum world which was enclosed and self-regulating (Goffman's 'Total Institution', 1961: 11). That the gatekeeper was a central figure in the running of the asylum was reflected in the 1819 Minutes of the Richmond Asylum, where a proposal was made and passed to provide a new great coat (National Archives of Ireland: Richmond District Lunatic Asylum Minute Book 1: 2.2.1819). The great coat as an item of clothing in the 1810s was essential for men and occupied an almost iconic place in nostalgic literature referring to out-of-date fashion by the middle of the century (Levitt and Tozer 1983 [2010]: 64; Sala 1859), when the great coat gave way to a lighter, slimmer overgarment (Burman 2003: 84). Sala stated in 1859 of the bygone fashion for great coats, that 'a new great coat was an event – a thing to be remembered as happening once or so in a lifetime' (1859: 59).

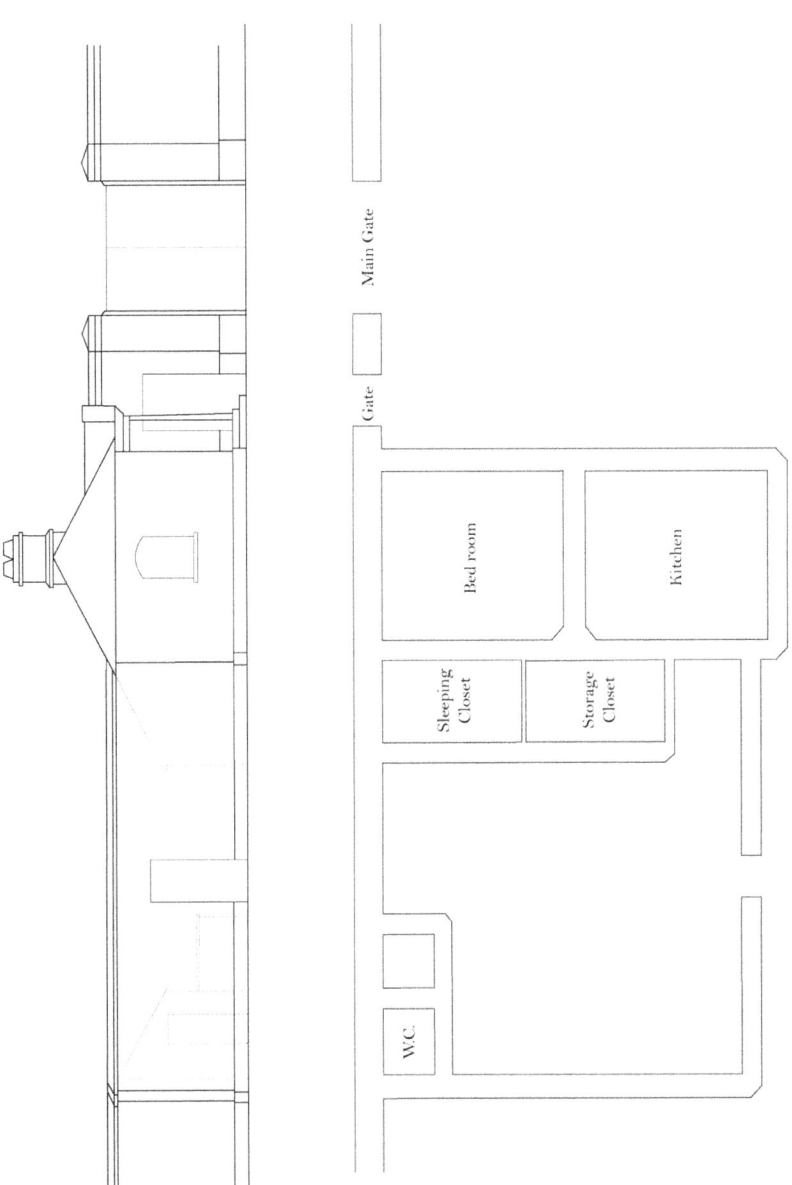

Figure 3.5 William Murray's schematic for the lodge at Maryborough District Lunatic Asylum (1830).

The provision of a new great coat for the gatekeeper at the Richmond Lunatic Asylum was a significant addition to his wardrobe, and also suggests that his previous attire was unsuitable. The provision of substantial additional, non-institutional clothing for a member of staff indicates that the gatekeeper was a critical component in the running of the institution, one for whom the provision of expensive garments was a necessity rather than a luxury. The separation of the gatekeeper from the general staff in status may have been intentionally stressed, as John Jacob states that the gatekeeper was responsible for controlling the access and egress of other staff, such as keepers, nurses, and servants.

The symbol of the gatekeeper's authority was his keys. Keys were a symbol of authority in domestic houses and other institutions in the nineteenth century (Pritchard 1991: 448; Vickery 2009: 43), as they represented the power of access and egress and also the power to inspect others. The gate and its lock were material indicators of authority and gravitas, as well as necessary security features. The gate installed at the main north gate of the Wakefield Asylum required the use (and bearing) of two keys which required simultaneous application in order to open (Stephen Beaumont Museum of Mental Health interpretive display). The gate was designed by lock makers C. Smith of Birmingham (after 1835, the company's foundation). C. Smith were a known supplier of prison cell locks and keys in the mid-to-late nineteenth century (Beck 2011: 7–8); the same may be said for Gibbons of Wolverhampton, who supplied the keys for the wings and cell doors at many other asylums, including the Irish provincial asylums. The Gibbons keys were stylistic in design and reflect a period of gothic-style key making. The use of large stylistic keys further reinforced the role of the key in the demonstration of authority and gravitas.

In his book about the Maryborough Asylum, Jacob listed note-keeping among the duties of the gatekeeper. The gatekeeper was to take notes on access to the asylum in a ledger (presumably housed at the lodge). The fact that this duty was explicitly mentioned in Jacob's book suggests that this passage was intended to contain a warning against collusion between the gatekeeper and the other staff members to move in and out of the asylum of their own volition (1833: 60). The clock atop the Maryborough asylum cupola was easily visible from the lodge, putting further onus on the gatekeeper to be accurate in his recording. He was answerable to the manager and matron directly. The architecture of the asylum and the gate lodge further reinforced both the gatekeeper's role and his status apart from the rest of the general staff. The Maryborough Asylum lodge offered a reasonable amount of private, separate space which only the manager's quarters surpassed. The lodge allowed for a reasonably sized bedroom, a kitchen, storage space, and a large yard to the rear. The gatekeeper at the Maryborough Asylum was expected to share his domicile with his wife. Given that the gatekeeper's domestic space served the dual purpose of domicile and office, the role of the wife in maintaining it was paramount. In the advertisement for a gatekeeper at Maryborough, the asylum asked specifically for a man with a 'clean wife', indicating the stress on maintaining an orderly internal space (Abbott 1833a).

The domestic and work space of the gatekeeper was within short walking distance from the asylum, with a clear view of the buildings. The lack of separation between the work and domestic space of the gatekeeper, and that of the other staff, further widened the gap between them. In the social hierarchy of the asylum, the gatekeeper's position placed him between the staff and the outside world, between the patient and the interior, and between the manager and the staff. Staff movements were expected to be accurately and precisely recorded by the gatekeeper, a small but alienating facet of his job. As a figure responsible for staff and patient movement and answerable to the manager and matron, the gatekeeper's position placed him in a liminal position in the asylum hierarchy. General staff and patients had to be granted permission to leave, most likely in written form. It is reasonable to assume that the gatekeeper had a reasonable degree of book-keeping ability, not to mention literacy; William Farrell of the Carlow Asylum wrote his memoirs while employed as gatekeeper. Modes of communication between the gate lodge and the main administration block were not standard for all asylums. Evidence from Maryborough indicates that the manager was in communication with the gatekeeper with regard to permissions for exiting the asylum, presumably inspecting his book. The carefully managed gardens of the asylums made the journey down the long avenue from the administration block to the gate lodge a journey of some gravitas. The approach to the asylum could be monitored from the lodge, actively or passively. As such, while the landscape around asylums was cultivated to provide a therapeutic aesthetic for patients to pass through, the watchful figure of the gatekeeper lent the main approach to the asylum building, and out of it, a panoptic air and a degree of respect reserved for management. As the first point of entrance and the last point of exit, the gate lodges and their keepers stood both inside and outside the asylum and represented a physical symbol of the power and authority of the asylum, and in turn the state or local government which supported it.

Government and asylum governance

The final section of this chapter will examine the influence of local or governmental authorities on the design and construction phase of asylum building in England and Ireland. The material examined in this chapter has focused on architecture, accounts, and ledgers. The accumulation of documentary sources for the period are considered here in the context of the role of asylums as mediators between the people and the state in the governance of the poor by local and national authorities. In the matter of governance, the asylum differed little from other public institutions, both despite and because of government insistence regarding the reform of asylums in the second decade of the nineteenth century. The influence of local and national government can be clearly seen in the portable material culture of the asylum, including the documentary evidence. Governance and the state in public asylums were particularly visible in Ireland, where the administration of asylums was, from the outset, an expression of (colonial) power. There were aspects of governance in nineteenth-century Ireland which shared commonalities with colonies in the British Empire. However, as part of the Union, Ireland was not strictly a 'colony', even if there were colonial elements in material culture and landscape.

The contested position of Ireland as a colonial territory within an empire, or an ethnic heartland within a broader British state, will be addressed here in the consideration of asylum governance as a national concern. Irish asylum governance will be compared with that of contemporaneous English examples of provincial institutions. Peter Bartlett has argued that the care of the insane in the nineteenth century cannot be separated from the development of Poor Law workhouses, stating that up to a quarter of England's lunatics were retained in workhouses following the 1808 Act (Bartlett 1998). I do not dispute this claim, but rather suggest that the Poor Law was a later feature of asylum development, which may be more relevant to the asylums constructed following the 1845 Act. The first decades of asylum administration following the 1808 and the 1817 Acts (in Ireland) were closely bound with local authorities and county councils, rather than national Poor Law commissioners.

The West Riding Asylum at Wakefield was, like other contemporaneously built asylums, constructed under the guidance of a local group of Visiting Magistrates and Visitors. This group was composed chiefly of doctors and landowners from the local area, working in conjunction with the local authority, following the 1808 Act urging the construction of asylums funded at county level (48 Geo.3 c.96; Levine-Clark 2004: 126; Snaith 1998). The Magistrates, based first at Pontefract and later at Wakefield, oversaw the development of the asylum from the planning phase through the formative years of development (West Yorkshire Archives Service West Riding: C85 1/1/1). This separates the Wakefield Asylum from those in provincial Ireland, whose construction was overseen by a government-appointed Board of General Control. Much like the Visiting Magistrates at Wakefield, the Board included four prominent doctors, various overseers of nearby institutions, and local landowners (National Archives of Ireland Commissioners for General Control: OPW 999/784); the difference lies in the remit of their duties. The Board of General Control were responsible for all of Ireland, whereas local groups like the Wakefield Visiting Magistrates were responsible for and to the Wakefield asylum alone, that is until the construction of a constituent institution at Wadsley near Sheffield in 1871 (Ellis 2008: 282). Until the introduction of the new Poor Laws in the 1830s, asylum administration fell under the remit of these local authorities, and administration was later undertaken by the Commissioners for Lunacy after the 1845 Lunacy Act. It is not until the construction of asylums on a large scale following the 1845 Act and the establishment of the Commissioners that bureaucratic documentation became standardised and formalised across Ireland and England, indicating a full administrative overhaul to cater for increased numbers and more centralised administration. Before 1845, apart from annual reports and quarterly accounts, asylums were relatively autonomous.

Dublin underwent a series of significant public works and civic improvement schemes in the late eighteenth and early nineteenth century. In addition to the construction of broad vistas and large public buildings, various bodies were set up at this time to oversee the redevelopment of the city. The Board of General Control was set up in 1817 following the construction of the Richmond Lunatic Asylum. The Board was to be responsible for the construction of four provincial asylums to support (and relieve) the asylums at Dublin and Cork. The Board was comprised of four doctors of medicine and the Director General of Military Hospitals, George Renny, among others (National Archives of Ireland Commissioners for General Control: OPW 999/784). This Board was the first step away from the homogenous institutional care of the poor, as the Board was dedicated solely to pauper asylums, setting those asylums apart from the Richmond Lunatic Asylum which was constructed under the eye of the local workhouse.

The first meeting of the Board of General Control took place in September 1817, attended by the members of the Board and representatives of the Lord Lieutenant, including Robert Peel. The minutes from this meeting are an example of the proceedings of the following two years. Peel in particular was concerned with the expense of four new provincial asylums, and on several occasions listed alternatives to the cost of hiring an architect and sourcing new building materials. Peel recommended the use of disused barracks no longer housing soldiers as well as the Roscommon Gaol, as mentioned earlier. Both alternatives were met with reticence by the Board, due to their unsuitability for use as asylums operating along the lines of moral management (National Archives of Ireland Commissioners for General Control: OPW 999/784, 27/9/1815; 15/12/1815). Much of the early meetings' minutes are taken up with responses to Peel's recommendations (which include hiring architect James Bevans, which will be discussed in the next chapter). Though little else is recorded, the rejection of Peel's recommendations suggests lively debate on the desired nature of a lunatic asylum, and a recognition that the patients of asylums were not to be treated punitively, as other institutional inmates.

While the treatment of lunatics within the asylums was intended to be focused towards the implementation of a more moral means of management, the placement of asylums varied considerably, suggesting less care put into the selection of a site than thoughts of convenience. The Maryborough Asylum, for example, was built on a site separated from a large convict gaol by a recently constructed road, and from the local infirmary by a redirected stream (Irish Architectural Archive Wilkinson Collection: 0085/138–116). The water source was, admittedly, an important drainage feature. William Murray's schematics of a pump house on the grounds and the redirection of the stream show that it acted as a water source for the asylum as well as marking out the site to the west; the deed for the land further indicates that the water was also a useful land boundary for the infirmary (Registry of Deeds of the Republic of Ireland: DI 865–184–58614). The proliferation of institutions in this undeveloped part of the Maryborough area mirrors the contemporaneous institutional 'district' in Dublin around Morning Star Avenue. The construction of the Lincoln County Asylum next to Lincoln Castle and near the city gaol echoes a similar desire to maintain an institutional locale to facilitate cooperation. As a consequence of the delegation of asylum construction to local authorities in the 1808 County Asylums Act, the lunatic asylum, like the local gaol or the workhouse, was a government institution by the nineteenth century. This relationship is more clearly marked out in some institutions than others.

The Richmond Lunatic Asylum in Dublin is a good example of a government-run institution. Instead of naming the asylum after the local area, the Richmond Lunatic Asylum was named in honour of Charles Lennox, Fourth Duke of Richmond and Lord Lieutenant of Ireland when the asylum was constructed. Lennox was a noteworthy figure, central to the political scene in Ireland and Britain in the first two decades of the nineteenth century. On quitting Ireland, Lennox moved his family to Brussels, where his wife held a ball attended by the Duke of Wellington – during which he was alleged to have been informed of Napoleon's advance towards Quatre Bras (Harvey 2007: 877–8)

– at which Captain Charles Verner, a relative of Johnston, was also in attendance (National Library of Ireland: MS/2722; Longford 1985: 230). Gifting the asylum and the adjacent penitentiary with his name fixed an association between these institutions and the power elites active in Dublin. The Lennox family crest and not the crest of the city or even Ireland was carved in relief above the door of the asylum. The Richmond Coat of Arms consists of a unicorn and an antelope (supporters) flanking a crested shield, topped by a crowned lion. The field of the coat of arms is divided in two and the shield is rounded (Burke 1832: 349–50).

The facade of Richmond Lunatic Asylum was not exceptionally decorated but for the relief carving of the coat of arms over the front doorway. The relief, positioned atop the lintel stone, stands out as the primary decoration on an otherwise unremarkable frontage. It is reasonable to suggest that the appearance of this sculpture above the doorway caught the attention of anyone entering the building. The mounting of an official coat of arms (with royal associations) on an otherwise unadorned building, directly above the entrance, suggests the intention of imposing an official government symbol on those who enter through the main doors. The heraldic symbol reinforced the authority of the material building. The Richmond Lunatic Asylum is a good example of how civic architecture used an expression of material power to maintain or justify the status quo (Pauls 2006: 66), in this case both in a social and governmental sense. The coat of arms represents the identity of not only the Duke of Richmond, but the established political elite in Ireland in 1815.

At other asylums, the association of the asylum with local and national governance was subtler. The iconography of the state was displayed on the portable material culture, for example the ceramic receptacles and platters used by patients and staff on all levels. The Maryborough Asylum plates and platters were stamped with a crown surrounded by a garter on which the asylum name was printed. This stamp imitates the 'Order of the Garter' stamp and suggests a firm declaration of the Maryborough Asylum as a government institution within the Queen's County (hence the crown) (Figure 3.6). The West Riding Asylum cups were also stamped with a garter, enclosing a rose and surrounded by a floral motif. The White Rose has been the symbol of Yorkshire since the fifteenth-century Wars of the Roses (Gore and Jones 2006: 137). These cups were common to all delegate asylums in the West Riding following the expansion of that system in the second half of the century. This style of imprint, utilising the county symbol, surrounded by a garter, was a standard symbol adopted in all asylum iconography. These ceramics were indicators of authority within the asylum. They are both composed

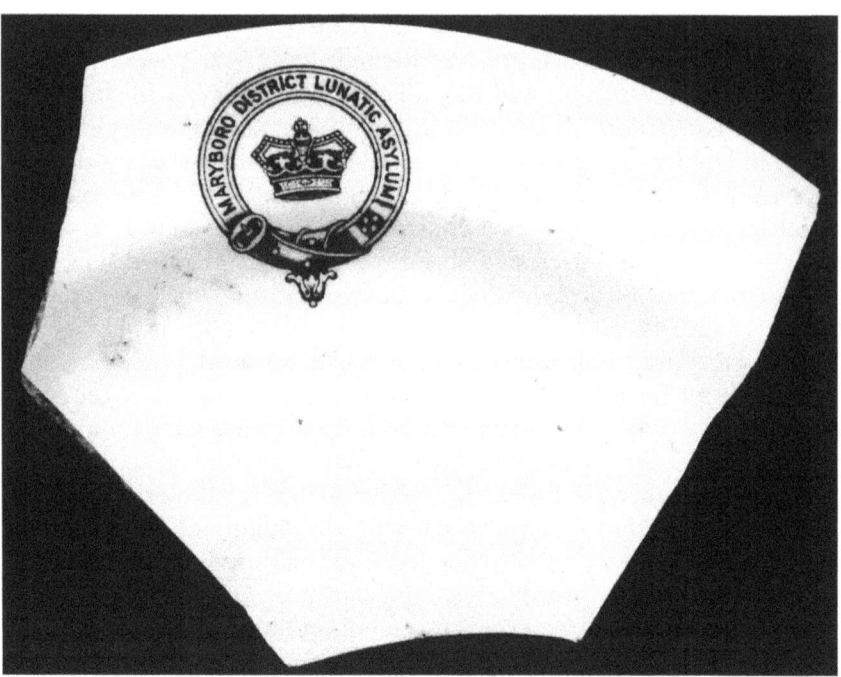

Figure 3.6 Platter fragment with Maryborough District Asylum stamp.

of strong, glazed earthenware and the lack of handle on the mug from the West Riding Asylum suggests that those mugs may have also been used by patients (a delicate handle may have been fragile).

Authority and bureaucracy in the historical record has been determined by use of minute books, ledgers, and accounts. These sources underwent changes throughout the nineteenth century, as discussed above with regards to administration reform. The sources also indicate social practice and habits. They evidence the sole use of English as the communication and administrative language in Ireland at this time. This feature sets the nineteenth-century sources apart from those of the twentieth century, following the separation of the Irish Free State from the United Kingdom. The quick adoption of Irish Gaelic (*Gaelige*) as an administrative language in the twentieth century may be seen as a postcolonial legacy of British rule in Ireland, and an exercise in the deconstruction of Ireland as a Union member. The following will consider the use of the English language at bureaucratic level in Ireland as a form of colonial-style dominance. The textual sources for administration in Ireland can be seen as material indicators of the homogeneity of the English language across the British Isles. The words and use of language evidence the audience for which the records were made, the education of the clerks, and the dominance of the English language over Irish in official parlance by the early nineteenth century. However, this may not be reflective of the patients or staff of the asylum. MacKinnon notes, in her assessment of asylum artefact collections in Australia, that the material remains of the asylums are silent: the cultural and ethnic diversity of asylum inmates is not reflected in the material culture. Equally, the range of languages spoken in the asylum is not reflected in that material either (2011: 86). Furthermore, the range of languages or dialects spoken at the case studies is not reflected in the textual material that remains from the asylums.

The number of people who spoke Irish in Ireland is disputed. At the start of the nineteenth century, the number of native and fluent Irish speakers (*Gaeilgeoirí*) has been estimated at 3.5 million. Its decline has been attributed to a series of factors such as the rejection of Irish by the Catholic Church, the English-language national schools (established in 1830), and the growing importance of English as a language tool for emigration (Miller 1988: 70; O'Néill 2005: 285). These figures testify to the decline of Irish as a written and spoken language. However, an 1812 source noted the difficulties in travelling through rural Ireland due to the dominance of Irish in the western counties in particular (see Wakefield 1812: 271, for example). The 1851 census returns indicate that of an overall Irish population of 6,552,386, only 23.3 per cent spoke Irish (The Census of Ireland 1856: xxvii). However, it must also be taken into account that the census date for 1851 was a Mothering Sunday (30 March). As such, many domestic servants working in urban centres such as Dublin may have been absent from the city that night, as tradition dictated that servants could go back to their parents on a Mothering Sunday (Shaw-Taylor 2007: 37). Therefore, some of the urban data may not be representative of the migrant working-class population inhabiting the cities on a daily basis. It is difficult to make assumptions based on the population data for this year, despite the fact that it was the first year when detailed questions were recorded with regard to education and trade.

The dominance of the English language in official administration and in the running of public institutions such as the Maryborough Asylum and Richmond Lunatic Asylum may have been an alienating feature for staff and patients. The dominant use of English reinforced the hierarchy in the asylum, which was topped by the manager and physician, who officially communicated in English. The rule boards composed for display at the Richmond Asylum (discussed in Chapter 2) were drafted in English, further reinforcing the idea that English was to be the official language spoken and displayed in the asylum, if not always understood in written (or verbal) form. The everyday tongue of general and support staff and patients (who were from a working-class or pauper background) is not reflected in the historical sources, but it was probable that Irish was spoken by many inside the asylums. Indeed, Irish may have been spoken as part of the maintenance of a clandestine economy among general and support staff, or among patients themselves. Irish may have been used as a linguistic and aural tool of resistance, much in the same way as it was used by female anti-treaty prisoners during the Irish Civil War who were confined at Kilmainham Gaol (Casella 2009: 180). Despite the fact that Irish was largely assumed to have fallen out of use in southern Leinster and Dublin by the mid-nineteenth century, the large amount of urban immigration, reflected in the demographic growth of Dublin, suggests that the population of Dublin may have been interspersed with native speakers from outside the city. Regardless, as the official administrative documentation for the Richmond Lunatic Asylum and the Maryborough Asylum were written exclusively in English, it must be assumed that Irish was not used in any official capacity. Irish may have formed part of the aural environment, though this is not reflected in the historical material.

National and local government and their associated agendas and private endowments were tied into the establishment and running of urban asylums such as the Richmond Lunatic Asylum. The Richmond Lunatic Asylum was bound closely with the political and social elite of Dublin at the time of construction, and with regards to the provincial Irish asylums, the influence of government is clearly seen in the involvement of Robert Peel during the planning stages. The Maryborough and Wakefield Asylums, as provincial asylums, utilised the symbols of their respective counties, demonstrating the close ties those asylums had with the local governments who were responsible for their financing. Despite the running of asylums as government institutions, however, it is possible to speculate on the presence of intangible modes of resistance within the asylums themselves, such as the use of different languages. This section has demonstrated the active role which national and local government had in the administration and management of public asylums. This can be considered an active attempt to associate with 'improvement', as in the case of Charles Lennox, and also as an exercise in exerting colonial influence on Ireland from the bottom, a necessary measure considering the status of Ireland as an antagonist in 1798 and as a recent addition to the Union.

Administration and bureaucracy

In this chapter, I have considered the process of facilitating and maintaining order in the asylum through a dedicated bureaucracy. The research conducted in support of this chapter indicated a shift towards standardised bureaucratic materials by the mid-nineteenth century. The asylum reports and accounts for Irish asylums from their opening until the mid-1850s were handwritten and contained limited personal accounts by the managers; reform in the administrative paperwork meant that following the 1850s it was printed and formalised. This demonstrated the centralisation of public institution administration in this period, which was marked by the change in paper-based records. This chapter also considered the architecture which utilised and housed the bureaucratic process, as well as the material culture of this process and the factors surrounding the administration of asylums. Gate lodges and administration blocks were the two primary foci of this chapter. Gate lodges were considered within the context of their stylistic correlations with country-house architecture. The gate lodges were examined as work spaces for the gatekeepers, who were considered a distinctive class in the social hierarchy of the asylum, set apart from the patients and lower-level staff by their association with authority and their duty as guardians of the asylum boundary. These buildings and their layout and staffing represented a link between the architecture of the asylum and that of the gentry, lending support to the assertion that asylum architecture was designed to reflect elite domestic architecture from the period.

The association with domestic and gentrified architecture was further reinforced by the administration blocks, which acted simultaneously as office, meeting, admission, and domestic space. The administration block of the Maryborough Asylum was a carefully designed building for efficient supervision and the inspection duties of the manager. The admission process was a physical and a bureaucratic ritual. In some cases, the admission spaces for patients were carefully segregated from the rest of the asylum, due to the necessity of carrying out various initiation rites to do with hygiene in particular. The design of the Wakefield Asylum was identified as effective in the execution of these rituals; however, the redevelopment of the Wakefield asylum may have altered these spaces, suggesting nuances in admission procedure beyond the standard process evidenced in the paperwork, such as the recording of names and illnesses, next of kin and age, signatories, and hygiene.

Clerical officers, as a distinctive group in the social hierarchy of the asylum, had a distinctive relationship with the asylum and other staff members. Their position was determined to be similar to that of the gatekeeper, as mediator between the general and support staff and patients and the upper-level management. Their occupations confined them to the administration space and material culture of the asylum so that they were separated physically, which reinforced the separation inherent in their position. Their position as keepers of the administrative paperwork also reinforced the separation between the clerks and the keepers, as their education and control over the paperwork placed them in a sub-management niche in the social hierarchy. The material culture of the clerical administration of the asylum demonstrates the responsibilities held by the clerical staff, as wielders of official insignia through stamps and wax seals, and also through inventories and records of items such as forks and ceramics. The stamps and numbers imprinted and painted onto asylum materials such as forks and plates were intended to act as deterrents to theft, consigning the clerks to the role of quarter-masters as well as administrators.

Stamps and insignias on plates and official asylum paperwork suggest a determination by the asylum to maintain officialdom in the operations of the asylum. This was lent to the material culture through the use of local and national authority symbols incorporated into asylum insignia, such as garters, flowers, and heraldry. These symbols implied ties between the asylum and local or national government which called forth the financing of the institutions by county authorities or by public figures such as Charles Lennox. The use of domestic architecture in the case of the gate lodge and the administration block demonstrates the social elevation of the people who were working inside, as well as supporting Tuke's notion that the asylum should be of a domestic style in order to downplay the institutional architecture. Spatial layout and written material indicate that the asylum was designed to create separate spaces for the specific use of management, clerical staff, and the gatekeeper. In the case of the latter two, the separate spheres and the records kept there reinforced their occupational responsibilities as sub-management. The use of English and the display of local and national symbols (or, in the case of Ireland, quasi-colonial symbols) demonstrated connections with government at these sub-management and higher management levels. The documentary accounts and material remains of the process of admission, management, discharge, and treatment remain among the most prolific records and material culture of the foundation period and early development of the asylums. I have highlighted the various architectural and spatial indicators which facilitated the maintenance and management of records, as well as determined the significance of symbols and language on the material culture and historical documentary evidence. In this manner, the rhetoric of reform inherent in the architecture and agents of bureaucracy and colonialism were compared with the record and material culture to determine practice.

4

Movement

> The building of a wall, the raising of a roof, the alteration of a door or window, or window-shutter, may materially affect the daily comfort of numerous patients, and the safety of others. What an anxiety for mere safety has suggested, may at once be seen by [the resident medical superintendent] to be inconsistent with light and cheerfulness, and apparent conveniences will to them always appear objectionable if purchased by a diminution of proper ventilation and warmth. (Conolly 1847: 7)

Hanwell physician John Conolly lamented the lack of consultation between architects and the resident or visiting medical men in public asylums. As an advocate of moral management, Conolly was concerned about the alteration of buildings and furnishings carefully chosen for reasons of moral, as well as physical, management. As discussed in Chapter 2, asylums like Hanwell (1831) were built and managed from the outset to reflect a more humane and caretaking attitude towards the mad. Features of this new generation of asylums included, variously, openable, paned windows and early attempts at central heating; these features were sometimes experimental and all developed by architects, or advised by reformers, with the view to creating a more moral asylum. As such, Conolly expressed concern that changes to the building, in the pursuit of convenience or security, altered those aspects of asylum spaces which were intended for the moral treatment of the patients as well as their physical comfort. Conolly was writing in 1847, when existing asylums were expanded to facilitate increasing numbers of patients and new asylums were planned or under construction. He was writing after the 1845 Lunacy Acts provided for the widespread construction of public asylums under the supervision of the new Commissioners for Lunacy. The care and comfort of the patients was, in Conolly's view, frequently set aside in the pursuit of a more efficient or more cost-effective asylum. The first chapter in this book examined the conflict caused by a difference in outlook between physicians and managers, and the ways in which the asylum building was designed and developed according to the demands of management and treatment needs. This was followed by an assessment of the uses of management space by figures outside traditional management structures, highlighting the role and influence of the country house and local and national government in the form and function of the public asylum. This final discussion chapter will build on the idea of experimentation and asylum-design-as-reform and focus on the physical spaces of the asylum and the creation and maintenance of prescriptive spaces for, in Conolly's words, light and cheerfulness, ventilation, and warmth. Surveillance and security were a primary concern of architects, doctors, and managers alike, and will be explored here with reference to one of the most common architectural principals attributed to asylum buildings, the *panopticon*.

Confinement was a facet of industrial life which, some have theorised, was necessary in order to maintain a social, industrious norm. In *Discipline and Punish*, Michel Foucault noted that the practice of individualising those who failed to conform to the expected standards of behaviour in an industrial city – i.e. those who could not or would not work – effectively homogenised the excluded, therefore creating a common and homogenous group identity among those bounded by exclusion from the everyday (2006). Foucault talked about asylums as part of a great Age of Confinement when, along with prisons and workhouses, asylums were developed to house those elements of society which did not conform to an industrious norm. The designation of abnormal – criminal, poor, insane – necessitated the creation of separate spaces in which these people could exist without negatively impacting the social norm. In confining large groups of abnormal, these groups themselves become homogenised. As such, the outside – the cities, towns, countryside, and public – may be seen as a heterotopia which the inmate must avoid in order to maintain institutional normalcy (Foucault and Miskowiec 1986). The heterotopia in the context of the lunatic asylum was unbound space, exterior to the consolidated common identity forged by the boundaries of homogeneity. In the lunatic asylum, the walls of the asylum, the enclosure of corridors, and the allocation of space for specific classified groups fulfilled the role of the 'utopia', while the outside world, from the perspective of an institutional life, may be seen or portrayed as unbounded and disordered, whose social norms were impracticable within the boundaries of the institutional utopia. Therefore, the material boundaries of the asylum may be seen to play an active role in the consolidation of order in the asylum building and the surrounding yards, gardens, and streetscapes. The buildings themselves represented the physical manifestation of moral management and were as much a therapeutic machine as contraptions for patient control like

William Saunders Hallaran's circulating swing. The creation of such an architectural machine was, in the early nineteenth century, a new concept for asylums, which had previously occupied the marginal and utilitarian fringe of architecture. The idea of the reformed moral asylum building had roots in a late eighteenth- and early nineteenth-century drive towards the creation of designated spaces for the 'other', as explored by Foucault, in which the asylum inmate may be cured and cared for away from the disruption of the increasingly industrialised city. The focus on cure and management, rather than confinement and restraint, resulted in several attempts by architects to design asylum spaces, from the smallest fixtures to the buildings themselves, for the safety and security of the inmate. The role of care in the creation of these bounded spaces must not be overlooked, even while care frequently took a backseat to expediency in the face of overcrowding or crisis.

Control and order were central to the mission and architecture of asylum buildings, just as they were in the prisons and workhouses which were designed and constructed at the same time. Though different in mission, asylum buildings owe a lot to other institutional buildings with which they frequently shared architects, patrons, land, and even inmates. The success of the architects' and reformers' mission to maintain control and order in increasingly large asylums is difficult to assess without analysing the physical space of asylums themselves. Archaeological approaches to historic landscapes have employed maps and plans to assess viewsheds (geographical areas visible from a location) (Delle 1998). Lunatic asylums, as large institutional buildings, were frequently constructed with viewsheds in mind – interior viewscapes which could be actively employed to prevent abuse and manage patient surveillance. Access and movement were central to management practices and a strict hierarchy of access was practised in asylums, with the manager or matron at the top, and confined patients and their visitors at the lowest levels. Employing graphical representations of the interior of a building showing permeability and pathways can illustrate the spatial hierarchy of the asylum as intended and devised by architects and managers. Access analysis maps – gamma maps – have been applied to asylum buildings in the past; as a method of spatial analysis, they were developed by architectural theorists Bill Hillier and Julienne Hanson (1984) and refined for the study of the spatial geography of the asylum by Thomas Markus (1993). Building on this previous scholarship, the graphical representation of access and hierarchy in the asylum will here be compared with the material world of the asylum, the materials and viewsheds enabled by or obstructive to ideals for reform and hierarchy.

Though not homogenous in shape, and significantly different in management and materials, certain shared features of asylum buildings will form the focus of this study, such as the approximate 1 m x 2 m 'cell' or patient bedroom, which appears on provincial asylum plans from the early nineteenth century and remained the norm for patient sleeping arrangements until the popularisation of the ward in the Victorian asylum in the 1850s. In the original designs of pre-1845 asylums, the spaces designed for the accommodation of patients were single-occupancy bedrooms. In some cases, patient rooms were required to house more than one patient – if necessary, up to fifteen people for short periods. The interior furnishings of the rooms consisted of at least one bed and a window. Room doors were generally perforated with a small hole for ventilation. Windows were usually located approximately 7.5 ft (2.3 m) from the floor level, with a rounded lower cill. Rounded cills in Irish asylums have been interpreted unfavourably as an oppressive feature and counter to moral management (Kennihan 2003). However, the construction of windows as such was likely to facilitate fresh air and light in the cell, without presenting a risk to patients intending to do him- or herself harm. The rooms were built to accommodate any patient type, and with a view towards high turnover in any case. The uniformity of asylum buildings makes them conducive to broad comparison between examples. This homogeneity has meant that nineteenth-century asylums are frequently homogenised as a single architectural form. During the early part of the nineteenth century, however, the new asylums constructed within the discourse of moral management, while sharing many common features with each other and with prisons and workhouses, were highly experimental. Principles for maintaining control of space were applied in multiple different ways. One such popular experimental feature trialled in asylums, prisons, workhouses, and other institutions was the panopticon, the architectural arrangement of a building to allow for maximum surveillance through centralised viewpoints and a radial design.

Panopticon, supervision, and the built environment

The panopticon was designed by British social reformer Jeremy Bentham at the end of the eighteenth century (1791). Bentham's panopticon, or Inspection House, was a theoretical architectural concept developed by Bentham and his brother for application to institutions where inspection and supervision were paramount. As an idea, the institution described by Bentham in his book, *Panopticon* (1791), seemed to answer a lot of the issues faced by eighteenth-century madhouses: supervision, staffing, and the negligence resulting from a failure of the former two. The mechanism of the panoptic building necessitated a large building with spacious cells and ample light. The position of the lodge at the centre of the cells, arrayed in a circle over two stories, meant that a superintendent or attendant might supervise all inmates at once, mitigating the problems caused by low staff numbers in public asylums in the eighteenth century. A lack of funding meant that public asylums in the eighteenth century operated with only a small number of staff. The panoptic principle could, theoretically, solve the problem of patient supervision, as well as facilitate the construction of lighter, airier asylums. For these reasons, Bentham's panopticon (1791) has been cited in secondary literature on the architecture of lunatic asylums as a primary influence in late Georgian design (Markus 1982, 1993; Smith 1999).

From an architectural perspective, asylums have been described as analogous with other contemporaneous institutions for confinement, like workhouses and prisons; Bentham thought that his panoptic design could be applied to any of these institutions to good effect (Bentham 1791: 2; Markus 1993). William Stark's 1810 design for Glasgow Asylum, a cruciform shape with four radiating wings and a central tower, demonstrates the early application of panoptic features in asylum buildings (Edington 2007; Smith 2007). In his own writing on the subject, Stark stated that his design would allow for those patients who were quiet and without need of supervision to be free of the imposition of active supervision on their daily lives. Equally, those patients inclined to misbehaviour or disorder would be aware of the unseen eye and would thus moderate their own behaviour (1810). He posited that while those who were in asylums were rarely acquiescent to their diagnosis, the patient's belief in the insanity of those around them would be sure to inspire appropriate behaviour under supervision. Stark's design for Glasgow was ambitious for the scale on which he was building, and heavily influenced by the reform writing he was (presumably) reading. He certainly visited the Retreat in preparation for designing the Glasgow Asylum, and spoke favourably of the furnishings of the building and the domestic nature of the asylum.

Taking the idea of patient classification seriously, Stark attempted to address the problems associated with mixing patients, expressing concern about the risk of violence or intimidation among the patients in the case of broad classifications. His solution was classification and spatial accommodation of patients in sixteen different groups in the asylum: two gender groups, a social rank division between higher and lower class, and within those groups a division of patients according to the severity of their condition: frantic, incurable, convalescent, and ordinary state. These patients were in turn to be distributed to different parts of the building, making their separate classification complete (Stark 1810). This complex classification system was to be applied in his panoptic-style building. However, despite the architect's confidence in his writing on the potential of a panoptic asylum design to moderate the behaviour of those within, the architecture of his asylum did not reflect a true panopticon; indeed, the very classification system he was intent on hindered the application of this relatively simple architectural principle. The design was difficult to put into practice, particularly given the security concerns associated with a lunatic asylum in a reformed system where the safety and security of a patient was paramount in a *de jour*, if not *de facto*, sense. Stark's design did allow for the internal observation of room corridors from keeper's quarters and for the observation of external yards from the first-floor keeper apartments, but his cross-shaped plan and circular central staircase made any lines of sight across the centre of the asylum impossible (Yanni 2007: 24). Furthermore, the day-to-day operation of the asylum, the movement of staff and patients, as well as the flexibility of routine were not taken into account. The success of a panoptic regime as described by Stark relied heavily on the maintenance of a strict routine and control of movement, on uniformity of behaviour and rigorous dedication to duty. The panoptic design, while elegant in its symmetry and facilitating of light and air in its long radial corridors, was not built to reflect the sometimes volatile and unpredictable nature of the people it housed; the open panoptic-style plan of the building meant that corridors were open on one side, reducing the effectiveness of patient classification as a means of noise control. The main fault with this system, though, was that it was far too tightly bound to the architecture of the buildings as they were designed. In his enthusiasm for a radial plan asylum, Stark had only provided for expansion along the lines of his cruciform original design; three of the four wings were added to before the asylum was finally converted into a hospital, and the asylum moved to Gartnaval on the north-west outskirts of the city in the early 1840s.

The success of Stark's Glasgow Asylum was heavily reliant on Bentham's central principle for the architecture, which was that behaviour hinged on the universal threat of observation from a central viewpoint (Bentham 1791; Semple 1993). The panoptic inspection house was intended to have the effect of total control through the threat of observation and presupposed the idea that the inmates of a panoptic institution would self-regulate when faced with the uncertainty of supervision from a vantage point (Casella 2007: 19; Foucault 1991: 202; Markus 1993: 123). The efficacy of such a system must be reconsidered in the case of a lunatic asylum, however. The moral management of patients entailed a minimal application of physical restraint in most of the asylums constructed after 1808. The pursuit of a restraint-free asylum drove many of the reformers of the period to open private asylums of their own in which to test their ideas, and several, such as

John Conolly, recorded and published their observations on the success of non-restraint (1847). The success of the system of non-restraint at the Lincoln City Asylum proved that it could be applied at a public asylum and was much publicised (Smith 1995). Minimal or non-restraint was certainly an ideal to which, by the 1830s, reformed asylum managers were expected to aspire. Non-restraint systems did not negate the need for an active management of patients through the physical presence of a superintending authority, not least as a precautionary measure against patient harm to themselves or others. However, in the ideal panoptic inspection house, supervision was hands-off, its success reliant on the idea that well-behaved inmates could self-regulate. As historical geographer Felix Driver has pointed out, the panopticon was inadequate as a reformatory model across all codes of institutions (Driver 2004: 11), due to the demands required in order for each institution – asylum, hospital, prison, workhouse – to operate as they were intended. The panopticon, a paranoia-inducing architectural mechanism, would be contrary to the aims of moral reformers of asylums, not least because it implied wrong-doing on the part of the patients and may have aggravated their illness. Physical surveillance and the presence of authority embodied physically by a keeper or nurse, at least during the day time, may be considered an alternative to the passive 'unseen eye'.

The practicality of surveillance, not only of patients but of keepers and nurses, was central to the planning of asylums. Prior to their construction, the West Riding Asylum in Wakefield and the provincial public asylums in Ireland were subject to competitions by architects for the design of the buildings. This was common practice in civic architecture of the period. Architects' designs were subject to scrutiny for effective use as lunatic asylums to be ideally operated under policies of moral management. In the instigation of a competition for the design of the Wakefield Asylum, the local magistrates had the competition advertised in regional and national newspapers, resulting in a variety of submissions (Figure 4.1). As discussed previously, the magistrates called on known asylum reformer Samuel Tuke of the York Retreat to advise particulars for prospective architects. Tuke made note of the need for 'vigilant inspection' of lower-level staff, in order to safeguard against abuse of patients by staff as well as to inspect patients and maintain good order. Tuke's concern for patient wellbeing at the hands of staff arose from the discovery of frequent abuse of patients by keepers at the nearby York Asylum at the end of the eighteenth century (Ashworth 1975; Tuke 1819). Tuke called for 'espionage' on staff to be taken on board. Espionage entailed an architecture within which the keepers could easily maintain surveillance on each other, on which they would be expected to report. Therefore, a vital component to the new

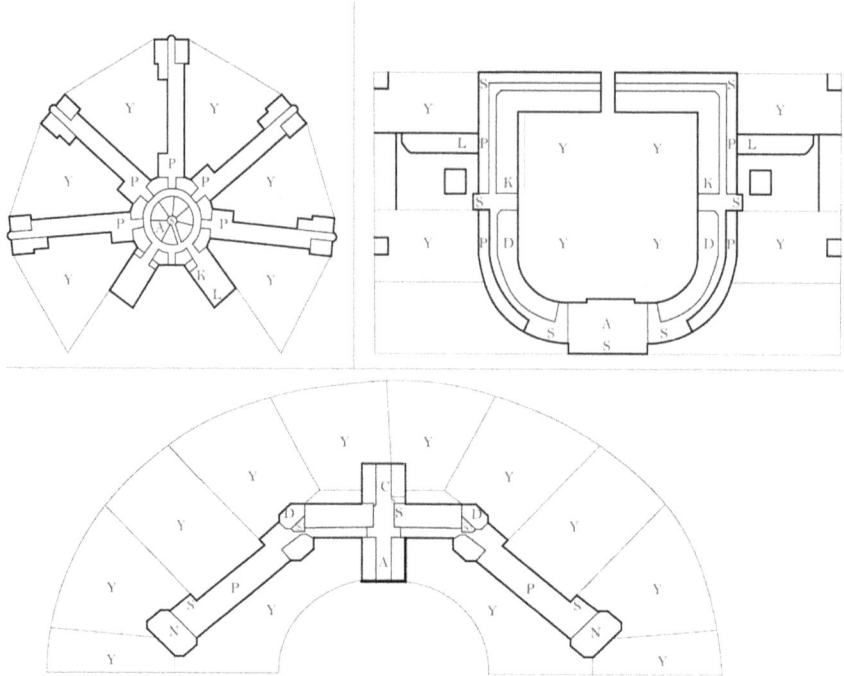

Figure 4.1 Submitted designs for West Riding District Lunatic Asylum. Clockwise from top right: Bevans' radial plan; Hainton's U-shaped plan; Lindley, Woodhead and Hurst linear plan. Administration (A), Convalescent Rooms (C), Day Rooms (D), Kitchen (K), Laundry (L), Noisy Patient Rooms (N), Patient Rooms (P), Stairs (S), Yard (Y).

Wakefield Asylum was to be that the keepers' rooms should be seen by each other. The inter-visibility built in to the asylum was to ensure the self-regulation of the keepers rather than the patients. For this reason, Tuke expressed a concern over the conversion of other buildings to the purpose of asylums (1819).

The specifications for the Wakefield Asylum ranged from practical considerations about water sourcing and ventilation, to concerns over the ability of the manager and matron to oversee their respective departments. The selection process concluded with the award of the contract to Yorkshire-based architects Watson and Pritchett. Their design topped a shortlist which also included London architect James Bevans and architects Lindley, Woodhead, and Hurst; both runners-up received recompense for their plans. Others in the running, but who were not awarded, were Hull architect Francis Hainton, whose application stated that he was 'hard up' and asked for consideration for runner-up to combat this (West Yorkshire Archives Service West Riding:

QD1/694); and two architects who submitted their designs under pseudonyms. One of these, 'Mediocrity', has been suggested to be James Bevans, due to the common address on documents in his file – 14 Grays Inn Square, London. However, this is unlikely as the handwriting and designs submitted by the two architects are significantly different. The other pseudonymous would-be architect styled themselves as 'Dum Spiro Spero' ('While I breathe, I hope' – Cicero). There are several possible candidates for this architect. Bethlem Royal Hospital have suggested that an architect of the same name for St George's Hospital, Southwark, was possibly John Gandy or James Gandon (Bethlem Royal Hospital Archives: YBP-22 M1/11). As there is a stylistic similarity in plan between the entrant to the West Riding Asylum competition and St Luke's Hospital, Moorfields, another possible candidate may be St Luke's architect George Dance Jr. However, due to Dance's advanced age at this time (he was 73), the architect may also have been his protégé, John Soane. Soane was a well-known antiquities collector, and the founder of a museum for his collection (Elsner 2004: 156; Furján 1997: 59). The use of a Cicero quote for the name may have been drawn from his interest in the Classics. Soane was interested in classical architecture, reflected in the design of his museum. An alternative to these architects is the suggestion that Dum Spiro Spero is no name at all, but a family or personal motto, and the plan is either anonymous or unsigned with accompanying documents lost. Incidentally, despite their lack of success in this particular competition, Dum Spiro Spero's plan was the closest realisation of Tuke's specifications. Table 4.1 illustrates each of the proposed plans for the West Riding Asylum, alongside a list of Tuke's specifications, many of which matched up with the didactic writing of other asylum reformers.

James Bevans's lack of success in realising an asylum design is interesting given his popularity at the time as a known asylum reform advocate. Bevans was a known Benthamite (Markus 1982: 97), and this is reflected in his panoptic-style asylum plans. Bevans was well known to Robert Peel, then Secretary to the Lord Lieutenant of Ireland, who recommended him to the Board of General Control in Ireland as a prospective architect for provincial asylums at the same time that he was compiling plans for the Wakefield Asylum. It may be a result of his notoriety as an architect, or his high friendships, that Bevans features so prominently in some of the literature of the period on asylum reform and architecture. Bevans's plans appear in House of Commons Reports, too (First Report 1815). His designs, though, never came to fruition. Bevans's famous design for a London asylum, with which he collaborated with architect William Hone, was shelved due to it being too expensive to build (Grimes 2008). A similar criticism is laid on Bevans

Table 4.1 Samuel Tuke's specifications for the West Riding Asylum, compared with plan features.

	W&P	JB-P	JB-L	L,W&H	FH	'DDS'	'M'
150 patients	Y	Y	Y	N	–	Y	–
Equal sex division	Y	Y	–	Y	Y	Y	Y
12 day rooms*	Y	N	N	Y	N	Y	N
8 courts	N	N	N	N	Y	Y	Y
8 galleries	N	N	N	N	N	N	N
Distinct sleeping rooms	Y	Y	Y	Y	Y	Y	Y
2 rooms for sick patients	N	–	–	Y	Y	Y	Y
Work room	Y	Y	Y	Y	Y	Y	Y
Committee room	Y	–	Y	Y	–	Y	Y
Apothecary shop	–	Y	Y	Y	–	Y	Y
Keeper accommodation	Y	Y	Y	Y	Y	Y	Y
Governor and Matron**	Y	Y	Y	Y	N	Y	N
Noisy patient accom.	Y	Y	Y	Y	Y	Y	–
Drying rooms***	–	–	–	Y	Y	Y	–
Laundry	Y	Y	Y	Y	Y	Y	Y
Brewhouse	Y	–	–	Y	Y	Y	Y
Bakehouse	Y	–	–	Y	Y	Y	Y
Bath	Y	Y	Y	Y	–	Y	Y
Designed to be enlarged	Y	N	N	–	–	Y	Y
Facility of inspection	Y	Y	Y	Y	N	–	N
Ventilated	Y	–	–	–	–	Y	Y
Brick building	Y	Y	Y	–	–	Y	–
Fire proof	–	–	–	–	Y	–	–
Diffusion of heat	Y	–	–	–	Y	Y	Y
Tanks for rain water	Y	–	–	–	–	Y	Y

Note: This table has been compiled utilising Samuel Tuke's *Instructions for the architects who prepared designs for the West Riding Asylum* (Tuke 1815, 1819), the architectural plans of the West Riding District Lunatic Asylum (Watson and Pritchett 1815; 1819), and the proposed drawings of the asylum (West Yorkshire Archive Service Catalogue: QD1/691-6).

Key: Y indicates that the plans/descriptions explicitly vouch for the presence of this room; N indicates that while the room/function exists, it is not of the same quantity or extent as the specifications provided by Tuke; – (null) indicates absence.
W&P: Watson and Pritchett (West Yorkshire Archive Service West Riding: C85/1355).
JB-P: James Bevans Panoptic Plan (West Yorkshire Archive Service Catalogue: QD1/691–2).
JB-L: James Bevans Linear Plan (West Yorkshire Archive Service Catalogue: QD1/691–2).
L,W&H: Lindley, Woodhead and Hirst plans (West Yorkshire Archive Service Catalogue: QD1/695).
FH: Francis Hainton Plans (West Yorkshire Archive Service Catalogue: QD1/ 694).
'DDS': 'Dum Spiro Spero' (*while I breathe, I hope*) plans (West Yorkshire Archive Service Catalogue: QD1/693).
'M': 'Mediocrity' Plans (West Yorkshire Archive Service Catalogue: QD1/696).

*   Overlooking the airing yards; 8 had distinct privies.
**   Must be placed to oversee respective departments
*** One male, one female; to allow for separation

NOTE: These observations were made based on the plans alone; no descriptions were enclosed.

by the Irish Board of General Control, leading to a less-than-civil correspondence between the Board and Bevans (National Archives of Ireland Commissioners for General Control: OPW 999/784). Bevans's designs represented an ideology of asylum and institution building, rather than a practical and viable option for those who held the purse strings. Still, his designs were innovative enough to warrant their consultation by Francis Johnston.

Six of the seven plans were accompanied by detailed written descriptions of how the building would function and how, if at all, they complied with Tuke's specifications. The top three designs were all enclosed in plan, allowing for maximum control of interior and exterior space, ensuring that the asylum was self-contained; surveillance is noted in each of the designs as a primary spatial feature. Bevans submitted two designs under his own name, and it is unclear for which one he was awarded second place and 70 guineas. One design was radial plan, while the other was linear. His linear design is a particularly good example of how surveillance was incorporated into the plans of these buildings as central feature of design. In the radial plan design, the manager's and matron's quarters faced into corridors and towards day rooms. However, in Bevans's design for surveillance, he was more concerned with the panoptic design feature of inmate surveillance, rather than the specifications recommended by Tuke: that the keeper's rooms should be arranged so as to promote self-regulation and peer management. Both Bevans's other design and his possible design under the name 'Mediocrity' are linear, early examples of this institutional style. Linear plans were favoured later by John Conolly in his 1847 book on ideal asylum architecture (Conolly 1847; Piddock 2007: 97). Linear designs placed the rooms of the manager and matron at the centre in the administration block, with little or no view of their neighbouring rooms and little view of the cells. Bevans's linear design, though promoting movement through the asylum and views from the ends of corridors, was presumably rejected on the basis of not having enough recreation space for patients and possibly on the issue of expense. Neither of Bevans's plans or descriptions noted the cost or means of ventilation, lighting, or furnishing.

The third-place design by Lindley, Woodhead, and Hurst placed keepers' rooms at the top of corridors, ensuring that patient corridors were surveyed but not allowing for easy movement through the asylum. Watson and Pritchett's winning plan (1819), by contrast, was H-shaped in plan. Their design consisted of two spiral staircases set in two octagonal towers from which the wings project, allowing staff members to traverse the stairs and gain floor-to-ceiling views into day rooms through grates over the doors; this shall be considered in more detail later. Watson and Pritchett placed the manager's and matron's rooms adjacent to the staircases, ensuring that they would be aware of movement up and down the stairs, as well as have easy access to them when supervision or surveillance was needed.

The Watson and Pritchett plan was similar to other lunatic asylums recently built in the British Isles, such as the Richmond Lunatic Asylum (1816). The Richmond Lunatic Asylum also showcased architectural expressions of contemporaneous ideas regarding the management of patients within an enclosed space. The enclosed space may have been seen as encouraging of the fostering of a domestic atmosphere among the staff and patients. Prior suggested that asylums placed an emphasis on the partitioning of internal space and the enclosure of the patient; partitions and boundaries are attributed to control and the maintenance of individuality (1988: 102). Rather (or perhaps additionally), this careful partitioning of space in the asylum may have been economic in motive. Tuke stated in his instructions to the architects that the drawbacks of private institutions were that they were commonly situated in previously occupied buildings and not built for the purpose of asylums. As such, the means of enclosing the patients with as few restraints as possible was not always realised. The lack of a large supply of keepers, or the capital to build a large, high wall meant that private asylums had a tendency towards insufficient attendance to patients, according to Tuke (1819). Therefore, the provision of a public asylum with large enclosing boundary walls broad enough to encompass gardens and yards enough for the maximum patient classification inside and outside would, on paper, necessitate fewer keepers and less direct physical restraint of patients. A building with an enclosed courtyard, self-contained in plan, was certainly that favoured in Ireland for its provincial lunatic asylums in 1817.

Concern over the reuse of existing institutional buildings and lack of suitable enclosed outdoor space was raised by Irish public works architect Francis Johnston in his assessment of the Roscommon Gaol for the purpose of a district asylum in 1817. Johnston's reservations were based on the lack of ventilation and ability for patient classification (National Archives of Ireland Commissioners for General Control: OPW 999/784: 16–18) in so limited a space, as discussed previously. Unlike at the Wakefield Asylum, Johnston's position as the architect of the proposed provincial asylums in Ireland read as a foregone conclusion in the minutes of the Board of General Control, who had charge of constructing an asylum system in 1817. Early in their planning, the Board asked Johnston and another architect – the (apparently) famous asylum architect Mr Bevans – to submit plans for two asylums, one for 100 patients and one for 150 (National Archives of Ireland Commissioners for General Control: OPW 999/784, 7; 25/9/1817). The Board's familiarity with

Johnston as the architect of several public buildings in Dublin, including several institutions, and engaged at the time in assessing Roscommon Gaol, meant that the Board passed Bevans's submissions on to Johnston for appraisal. Their aim in doing this was to engage Johnston to design an asylum based on his comparative scrutiny of the plans – Mr Bevans's and his own. Johnston's original design, or the design assumed to be such (Johnston 1817 – St Patrick's Hospital Archive Plan No. 2: F/6), was not very different from Bevans's radial asylum design for the West Riding Asylum, or indeed William Stark's Glasgow. More baths and rooms were added to the working plans of the provincial asylums, plans which directly resulted in the construction of Armagh District Asylum for 100 patients in 1828 and Limerick District Asylum for 150 patients in 1827 (Lewis 1837). Considering his plan of the proposed London asylum, and those he submitted for the asylum at Wakefield, the plans which Bevans submitted were probably both radial and linear in style (as per West Yorkshire Archives Service Catalogue: QD1/691). Bevans was extremely put out that his plans were shown to another architect, and his correspondence with the Board of General Control ended abruptly in 1817.

There are several variations of Johnston's plan for provincial asylums in Ireland. One unlabelled plan in the Irish Architectural Archive was discovered in Belfast Lunatic Asylum, showing a similar but not identical asylum plan to that constructed at Belfast. The plan is a minor variation on Johnston and Murray's plans for a K-shape 100-patient provincial asylum and is evidence of a degree of experimentation in how these buildings were designed. The cupola atop the provincial asylums is present in this draft and suggests a later date for this unidentified plan, but may still indicate the progression of Johnston's design concept. The final plan executed for the Irish provincial asylums for 100 patients was linear in style with radial projections and incorporated the changes that Johnston made to the original following his examination of Bevans's plan. Johnston's original cruciform design, and the resulting X-shape asylum plan, were enclosed in form. While this conformed to the desired design, it also allowed for continuous movement through the asylum wings. Movement was hindered by doors at the ends of corridors, though all were interconnected. A high-level staff member, such as the manager, could access all parts of the asylum without having to retrace his steps. The lines of sight in these corridors allowed an authority figure unhindered access to the end of their corridors. The fact that the cell doors were all on one side of the wall allowed the patient within a certain degree of isolation. Their door was not facing another patient's room. Johnston's design incorporated moral management principals, as well as a degree of panoptic-esque features, though it cannot be said that his designs were strictly panoptic.

Johnston died in 1829, leaving the provincial asylum system in Ireland still unfinished. His designs were taken up and improved upon by his protégé and nephew William Murray. Even so, there is only limited variation between the first asylum at Armagh (1825) and the last to be built at Waterford (1835). Architectural historian Ryan Kennihan has suggested that the panoptic 'ocule' in Johnston and Murray's provincial asylums was indicative of the presence of a manager in residence in the administration block (2003: 54). Rather, it is probable that this 'presence', instead of representing an oppressive authority figure, was intended as a reinforcement of the principals of moral management – specifically the idea of the asylum as a 'domestic' institution. This idea was encouraged by reformers like Tuke (1813). The manager of Johnston's provincial asylum was indeed afforded a view into the internal courtyards from his rear domicile windows, though the elevation of the building indicates that the windows are wide and tall, making any supervising eye visible to those outside. As such, any authority figure would not be unseen. Further to this, the working plans of the Carlow District Asylum label the internal courtyard as the 'Governor's Yard' (Irish Architectural Archive Murray Collection: 0092/046–0412). It is unclear what the function of the yard was; the staff hierarchy of the asylum suggests that the 'Governor' was in fact referring to the manager who was resident in the building overlooking the yard. The distinctive labelling of this yard as the 'Governor's', rather than Airing Yards, suggests a specific purpose apart from the day-to-day running of the asylum. The Governor's Yard may have been reserved for specific patients; for example, fee-paying patients.

Kennihan's (2003) suggestion that the Governor's (manager's) house holds a central position as a surveillance point may be considered in another way: the manager's house was accessed by a central staircase, granting him entry to the administration block and the primary approaches to the lateral wards. Staircases to either side of the house, down to access corridors in the lateral wings, allowed the manager to have private ingress to different parts of the asylum. Keeper behaviour and the proper management of the asylum could be regulated by the threat of the manager's appearance at any time; this may not have had any effect on the patients, but may have policed keeper behaviour. As a result of these staircases, the wings effectively became a controlled, bounded space, where actions were accountable to a mobile authority figure whose points and directions of access were multiple.

Despite the influence that Bentham and his panoptic plans had over institutional design, the panoptic plan for lunatic asylums was disregarded by asylum designers in the second half of the nineteenth century, in a move away from the association with prison architecture

(Carpenter 2010: 60). Regardless of the influence of Benthamite asylum architects, and the ideological popularity of the panopticon, the finished designs of lunatic asylums in this period were more actively concerned with the control of interior space through physical barriers, though the architecture of the buildings incorporated certain panoptic features to cultivate an institutional, or at least a civic, aesthetic. This suggests that management of lunatic asylums in this period was primarily based on physical obstruction and active patrolling, rather than the omnipresent threat of perpetual surveillance.

The original Richmond Lunatic Asylum in Dublin consisted of an administration block with two lateral wings, connected to the rear by a corridor, enclosing the interior space and connecting the wings to the utility block. In the decades following construction, a central corridor system divided the interior courtyard of Richmond Lunatic Asylum into a quadrangle. This corridor system – which was restricted to the ground floor alone – separated the central courtyard into a quadrangle, dividing patients of pauper class from those of higher class (Irish Architectural Archive Murray Collection: 0092/046–0412). The division of the interior yards also had the effect of separating male patients from female patients. The plan of Richmond Lunatic Asylum complete with the central courtyard bears resemblance at first glance to plans for a Benthamite penitentiary by Bevans, which consisted of a central observation tower surrounded by concentric cells. It should also be noted, however, that the central octagonal structure where the corridors of the quadrangle met had too few windows to operate as an observation centre and was in any case on the ground floor only (Irish Architectural Archive Murray Collection: 0092/046–0412; 0092/046–0421; 0092/046–0422). The octagonal structure at the centre of the corridor system was intended for use as a utility block, housing sculleries and boiler rooms. The original plan of the building was to include a kitchen and utility block at the centre of these corridors; this was deemed 'unnecessary' by Johnston as early as October 1814 (Irish Architectural Archive Murray Collection: 0092/046–0411). The corridor facilitated convenient access for staff members to all parts of the house. The asylum plan indicates that the central octagonal hallway at the crux of the bisecting corridors could not practically be used as an observation centre, though it was in the most convenient location for one. That it was not used as such indicates that observation from a central vantage point was not a priority for Johnston or the Board in the intended management of the asylum.

From the central crux, any views to the east and west along interior courtyards were obscured by staircases with a central dividing wall. To the south, the observer would be afforded a view into the entrance hall, to the front door. To the north, the line of sight offered a view towards the kitchen block, likely obstructed by doors. No views of cells were possible from the central structure, internally or externally. Corridor observation was therefore delegated to keepers occupying the offices at the ends of each corridor. Keepers and nurses would be required to move around the corridors in order to maintain active surveillance. It is more likely, therefore, that patients were left to their own devices when in their cells and keepers were not required to survey them at all times. Given the expense incurred in maintaining a panoptic system of surveillance, it is unlikely that this system was ever implemented in the long term in public asylums.

The plan for the Wakefield Asylum incorporated passive surveillance in a novel manner, as per Tuke's instructions and his emphasis on maintaining order among the keepers. Watson and Pritchett provided for views into patient day rooms with the construction of two octagonal towers at the intersections of their H-plan, in which the governor and matron were housed and from which patient corridors could be accessed. These towers allowed for easy access to the central corridors which connected the male and female sides of the house (Markus 1982: 97). Spiral staircases facilitated movement up through the towers and were installed with intermittent 'bird nests' – recessed landings. These bird nests allowed a keeper or management figure to stand on the stairs at strategic points and observe day rooms through windows over their doors (Ashworth 1975: 17). The architects envisioned a view into day rooms from floor to ceiling from the vantage points of the nests. Movement up and down the stairs would allow for a view into day rooms on either side as the stairs were climbed. The staircases lead to an octagonal room in the attic, with windows that faced out over the grounds.

The architect's elevation of the octagonal towers illustrates that the room at the top of the stairs could not be used as any kind of observation centre for the yards outside, and indeed the windows were almost too high to afford a view out. Furthermore, the windows in the tower faced out over the roof of the asylum, rather than into any of the internal or external yards. The room at the top of the stairs could be used as a place to turn and descend, suggesting that active movement from one station to another was more important than passive, unmoving supervision. The galleries could also be used for patient exercise. The bird nests indicate that unimpeded supervision was considered in early nineteenth-century asylums. While supervision was certainly possible, though, it does not discount the possibility that anyone on the stairs could be both seen and heard through the grilles set above the doors. While similar to the panoptic style of management, the authority figures in this case played a more physically and visually active role in the supervision of patients.

The difference between an unseen entity supervising goings on and the certainty of supervision is visibility and security, for the patients as well as the staff. The 'unseen eye' and an emphasis on isolation could have a potentially damaging psychological effect on inmates in prisons (Tarlow 2007: 136), and the installation of such a system in a lunatic asylum therefore could not have been practical. Indeed, it would have been contrary to moral management practice. The benefit of the certain knowledge of a physical presence, either through their visibility, sonic presence, or physical interaction, is the reduction of isolation.

The level of access assured the managers of the provincial Irish asylums supports the assertion that movement, rather than observation, was central to the running of asylums. While keepers and nurses were afforded views of the corridor from one end, it was not possible to adequately survey all patient room doors from one central position. The layout of the corridors (Irish Architectural Archive Murray Collection: 0092/046–0137) does not support there ever having been a central observation point; rather, much like their predecessor the Richmond Lunatic Asylum, each corridor was enclosed. In this manner, the keepers and nurses were responsible for the ordered maintenance of the corridor and the supervision of patients, under threat of visitation and inspection by the manager themselves. A panoptic influence may be attributed to the cosmetic design of the provincial asylum exteriors. The tall cupola which stands over the administration block housed a clock, implying order and regulation of time in the institution. In the plans, there is no indication that the cupola was used for surveillance, though this may not be discounted.

Murray's elevation of the provincial Irish asylum cupolas was annotated to suggest that shutters on the side of the tower may be adjusted open or closed (Irish Architectural Archive Murray Collection 0092/046–0132). However, rather than acting as an imposing 'ocule', the cupola may rather be seen as a symbol of asylum – and civic – authority, lending a degree of austerity and institutional power to the building when viewed from outside, as well as serving as a reminder to those viewers inside of authority within. The cupola as an architectural indicator of power and the panoptic gaze has been suggested by Leone in his study of historic Annapolis; he suggested that the cupola drew the eye of those inhabiting the space around it, thus drawing their eyes to the authority of the state (1995: 257). Johnston's cupola, as well as Watson and Pritchett's octagonal towers, may not act in practice as panoptic apparatuses, but their role as power statements – in that they draw the eye of the observer – was more effective in communicating power and authority than in actively engaging with it.

Despite the myriad features attributed to the influence of Bentham in the asylum, the panoptic gaze was not practicable within the existing architecture, though it may well have dominated the ideology. The architecture of asylums hints at an influence by Benthamite designers. Bevans's notoriety as an asylum designer despite his meagre catalogue of works demonstrates the popularity of panopticism as an ideology, if not in building or preferred design practice. Indeed, while asylums may not have operated on the principle of panopticon, their architecture demonstrates a physical influence and even an attempt to seem panoptic even if they are not. The Wakefield Asylum's towers, for instance, appear to the observer as possible observation towers on a cursory glance; however, closer inspection shows that their ability to function as such was hindered by the fact that the windows of the tower faced out over the rooftops, rather than into the courtyards. The cupolas at Maryborough and Carlow District Asylums, while offering a focal point for the architecture and stamping the presence of the asylum on the townscape, were not practically operated as panoptic features despite the potential to do so. Panopticism may therefore have featured in asylum architecture as an aesthetic, rather than management, feature. Towers, for example, may lend a degree of gravitas to a building, particularly one that is built to fulfil a utilitarian purpose, and to discourage people not in need of the asylum's services from making unnecessary use of the institution.

In their notes on the outward appearance of the Wakefield Asylum, Watson and Pritchett stated that they, as well as the magistrates, were mindful that 'the building was a Pauper Asylum', and further pointed out that a great deal of care was made to incorporate functionality into any architectural decoration, such as cornices made into gutters (1819: 30). The concern appears to be in maintaining a degree of functionality, so as to demonstrate the practical running of the asylum which was partially funded by the public purse. Thus, the asylum was constructed to reflect internal practice and management according to practicality.

Other physical attributes associated with asylum design in the nineteenth century were single patient rooms, heavy doors, and large sets of keys. In turn, historic asylum buildings are frequently associated with mechanical sounds and dim light. Museums and collections frequently display large locks, isolation cells, and other material indicators of power and incarceration. Two of the most common artefacts displayed from asylums are keys and locks. In museums, these are arrayed in cases or hanging from large rings worn by mannequins dressed as keepers. The display of such items suggests that 'locking' the asylum was central to the running of the building and the internal atmosphere associated with it. However, the role of the lock and key in the practice of moral management must be considered with a view to the care as well as the confinement of the patient.

Tuke's emphasis on the creation of a 'domestic' institution in his descriptions of his own asylum, the Retreat (1813; Yanni 2007: 27), is symptomatic of the growing divide between physical and psychological medicine in the early nineteenth century. Unlike the development of hospitals for the sick, and prisons for the unruly, the lunatic asylum was emphasised in early didactic literature as a portrait of domestic life, further reinforcing domestic class divisions and emphasising social order (Markus 1982: 106; Yanni 2007: 24). The parental roles of the manager and matron further testify to this. The matron was responsible for visiting every female patient once a day, for example (Bolton 1928). Whether or not these duties were carried out, the description of these roles in didactic literature demonstrates that the asylum was intended to function as an ordered domestic household. Keys were indicators of authority in Georgian Britain, as were access privileges (Vickery 2009: 43). As such, keys were rationed within the Georgian household; they were generally entrusted to a few people, though domestic keys were generally under the ownership of the head of the house (Vickery 2009: 42). Keys in asylums were, in turn, limited in circulation and distributed discerningly. Movement through corridors of cells was the reserve of the keyholder, and the securing of patients in rooms was vital to the maintenance of order in the house. Buildings and architectural layouts have an effect on social interaction (Gieryn 2001: 46). Therefore, the creation of these corridors of individual sleeping rooms for patients contributed to the creation of a stratified hierarchy. The relationship between patients and keepers or nurses was defined by a power structure based on key possession and access. The keys made noise, especially when hanging from large loops attached to the uniforms of keepers and nurses. The sonic presence of a keeper within the corridor may have lessened the sense of isolation inbuilt in a single patient room. There may have been active intention to imbibe a sense of secure and parental presence immediately outside the rooms.

Social meaning can be written into the sonic properties of architecture, fostering an interior atmosphere that can affect behaviour (Blesser and Salter 2007). The effect of sound must therefore not be discounted in the construction of habitable spaces – as the domestic asylum was to be (for further discussion of the sonic environment of Georgian lunatic asylums, see Fennelly 2014). In the 1830s, Maryborough-based physician John Jacob remarked on the effect of noisy patients on convalescents:

> let anyone who has ever seen the interior of a lunatic asylum, consider within himself what chance there exists that the poor convalescent should, in his hours of recovery, hear the conversation likely to lead him back to wise and happy thought. The presence of a company of

lunatics, their incoherent talk, their cries, their moans, their indescribable utterances of all imaginable fancies or their ungovernable frolics and tumult, can have no salutary effect on a mind just recovering from long depression. (Jacob 1833)

This demonstrates a concern over the effect of one patient's illness on another with regard to the amount of noise they made, and the internal atmosphere of the asylum as a place of therapy. His commentary – relating specifically to the Maryborough Asylum – illustrates the atmosphere of the asylum, representing the building as noisy and busy.

The cultivation of an atmosphere, as well as an appearance and routine of domesticity, was applied to the allocation and classification of patient rooms. Tuke, for one, was concerned with the careful separation of rooms for 'noisy patients' and recommended to the prospective architects of the Wakefield Asylum that noisy patient rooms be situated in the building to cause the least amount of disruption (1819). Watson and Pritchett's plan provided for refractory patients in the north wings of Wakefield Asylum. In his 1816 plans for the Richmond Lunatic Asylum, Johnston also made a provision for the accommodation of convalescent (recovering) patients in a separate wing of the asylum, which was planned to be constructed so as to physically connect the asylum with the Whitworth Surgical Hospital. This connecting wing was to face the western gate of the asylum, which in 1816 looked out onto farmland (Irish Architectural Archive Murray Collection: 0092/046–0183). Though Johnston's new wing was never built, it does indicate a conscious effort to accommodate patients according to the beneficial effects of the internal sonic environment: convalescent patients, in recovery, could benefit from removal away from noisy patients and corridors to a quiet outlying wing.

Designs of locks, doors, and windows were a common feature of architects' plans. Architects were responsible for interior fixtures such as bolts, and their design was to reflect moral management as much as any exterior architectural feature. In their original notes, for instance, Watson and Pritchett stated of the Wakefield Asylum that, 'there are no bolts to any of the patients' rooms: the doors are secured by strong half mortice locks, of a very simple construction, suggested by the Clerk of Works at the York Asylum: the result of his observation on the inconveniences and expense attending the common locks' (1819). Though the architects do not state whether they are referring to solitary confinement cells, the omission of bolts may have had another motivation. Tuke notes in his description of that asylum that the doors of the Retreat were equipped with a spring mortice lock and a bolt, though the sound of the bolt drawn on the doors of patients' rooms at the Retreat was a cause of some objection, and that the spring mortice lock sufficed. The objection that Tuke raised to the bolts was noted by William Stark when he visited the Retreat before designing the asylum at Glasgow. Stark remarked that the managers, during his visit, were occupied with discovering a solution to the bolts on the doors, whose 'harsh, ungrateful' sound put them in mind of a prison (Stark 1810). Tuke himself notes the 'grating sound' in his own book three years later (1813). It is noted later in the nineteenth century that asylum door locks were encased in leather, to muffle the sound of the bolts (Laffey 2003: 1293). This suggests that, among other derivations from the Retreat, such as iron bed style (West Yorkshire Archives Service West Riding: C85/1/1/1), the bolts were omitted from the doors of Wakefield Asylum in favour of the mortice lock. Conversely, Johnston and Murray's patient room doors were illustrated with a large bolt and a padlock; there is no evidence that any attempt was to be made to muffle the sound (Irish Architectural Archive Murray Collection: 0092/046–0128). This suggests that the architects did not take the effect of the locking sound into account, demonstrating a lack of consultation with contemporaneous asylums in England which were being built for reform, such as the Middlesex, Lincoln, and Wakefield asylums.

The development of the padded cell in the later nineteenth century reflects a lack of success on the part of the architect in creating a wholly separate space for noisy patients. It also suggests developments in the consideration of classification: the creation of a separate isolation cell specifically for the noisiest or most unruly patient reflected a lack of classification in practice such that an exceptional measure was necessary. The Stephen Beaumont Museum of Mental Health in Wakefield houses a complete solitary padded cell, as does the small collection for the former Richmond Asylum, albeit in a more ruinous state. Separate padded cells were common in asylums by the end of the nineteenth century. Certainly by 1897 there were at the Cork Lunatic Asylum, with a call for more (The Forty-Seventh Report 1898). The cells were lit by a small window in the door, which acted as both a viewing panel and a means of letting light in. The cells for the Wakefield Asylum and at the Richmond Lunatic Asylum in Dublin were both manufactured by the Pocock Brothers, putting the date of these specific cells to the period around 1902 when the Pocock Brothers, suppliers of asylum-specific apparatuses, showcased their 'padded rooms for institutions' (Anonymous 1902). The Pocock Brothers represented an industry, advertised in journals such as the *British Medical Journal*, dedicated to the invention of objects and machinery for use within the medical and mental health services. This dedicated industry suggests a level of refinement and sophistication in the treatment of patients by the end of the nineteenth century, and a movement away from the architect as a primary influence in the running of the building. The Pocock Brothers' door and cell design on the early twentieth-century padded cell demonstrates a movement away from concerns about the noise of bolts over time. As with the architectural arrangement of the asylum, the idealism that saw the omission of bolt locks from the patient room doors when the asylum was founded was omitted later, whether in favour of practicality or economy; neither are clear motivations.

Creating a solution to the problem of institutional sounds by encasing locks and omitting bolts also indicates a lack of account, on the part of the asylum authorities, architects, and idealists, for the day-to-day running of the asylum. The actions of the keepers and nurses, and their presence in the corridors, generated acoustic indicators of authority which were not deadened by the building. The experience of the patient in the asylum was deemed as comfortable due to the omission of a loud, institutional noise: the bolt on the door. However, though the moderation of institutional sound had minimal effect and could not be counterproductive to the other components of life in the asylum, sound and acoustics were a concern in the design process. The internal acoustics of the Irish provincial asylums have generally been concerned, as Dr Jacob was, with patient noise and classification according to unruly or noisy behaviour rather than the built environment constructed to reflect such noise, as well as the background sounds of the running of the asylum.

Vaulted ceilings were a common feature of asylums in the early nineteenth century. At the Wakefield Asylum, the patient room ceilings and corridors were vaulted, while offices had flat arches. The vaulting of ceilings in cells may indicate an awareness of the acoustic properties of the building technique and the usefulness of this technique in containing patient room and corridor noise. A convex ceiling focused sound, rather than scattering it, minimising the number of surfaces against which the sound could bounce (Brown 2008: 29–30; Moore 1967: 20–3). This was hampered somewhat by the convex window cills common in Irish provincial asylums, which could scatter sound throughout the room, though the small surface area would limit the effect. Patient room window cills were generally rounded. The purpose of the rounded cill in the cells was safety: light was still able to penetrate into the patient rooms.

Floor covering – an essential feature of a domestic asylum – is rarely recorded in any detail in the documentary record. Elevations of selected asylums including the Irish provincial asylums indicate that upper stories had floor boards, along with the ground floor storey above the basement. Maryborough District Asylum's basement was flagged, as was the ground floor where the basement did not extend. In his plan of Carlow District Asylum, Murray explicitly stated that the basement storey be flagged with a channel cut in the stones of the rear passage

(Irish Architectural Archive Murray Collection: 0092/046–0123). This channel would have ensured that the bath in the basement could overflow without flooding. There is no channel cut into the Maryborough District Asylum basement corridor flagstones, but a channel may have been cut into the patient rooms or bath floors on that level. Regardless, Murray's explicit statement of materials suggests that there was a consciousness of the properties of materials used on the part of the architect and the Board which approved plans.

A wooden surface, as a porous material, would allow for absorption of noise (Moore 1967: 27), though a flagged surface may not. The porous nature of limestone, the material with which the Maryborough District Asylum was constructed, may have allowed for absorption of some sound, though the vacancies caused by the vaulting to support floors on the upper stories may have allowed for more reverberation and low-level sound, despite the absorbing properties of the wood. The angular ceilings of the Richmond Lunatic Asylum would have reflected sound from the corners, creating an echo (Moore 1967: 23). The effect of this on the patients, or on the containment of patient sound within a cell, may have influenced Johnston and Murray's decision to design the Irish provincial asylums with vaulted ceilings. In the Wakefield Asylum, the ground floor rooms were flagged, while the upper-floor rooms were boarded. The architects noted that the northern end of the wings contained rooms for 'violent, noisy and dirty' patients, with floors consisting of a 'single flag' with a drainage channel. The use of a single flag may have minimised noise dispersal; noise may be dispersed through breaks in a surface, such as gaps between flagstones. The use of a single flag was likely intended as a sanitary and safety measure, and the favourable acoustic properties were a useful coincidence.

The control of sound and acoustics indicates that the complete control of the interior environment, as well as sensory control, was central to the planning of an asylum at this time. This supports the assertion of sociologist Erving Goffman that an institutional environment, removed from the space and environment of the outside world, would institutionalise the patient and allow for the maintenance of control and order (1961: 24). However, where Goffman's work focuses on the debilitating and demoralising effects of this institutionalisation of the patient, the intentions of the architects and planners of the early lunatic asylums may be seen as care-driven. Goffman equates asylums with prisons and concentration camps and treats all as 'total institutions'. Each institution focuses on the physical and mental control of the inmate, though as demonstrated by Tuke's concern for patient experience, the lunatic asylum and the planning of interior space and environment for these institutions may be said to reflect a certain duty of care to patients. As stated by Australian historian of medicine Dolly MacKinnon, madness cannot be said to be 'silent', and the patients' 'interior soundscapes' – the noises of their own heads – affected their treatment and classification; therefore, their perception of their own environment through sound was vital to their management and treatment. Concern over how soundscapes affected patients, and the subsequent measures taken to minimise institutional sounds, reinforced the idea of care in the asylum's sonic as well as spatial layout.

The design of asylums and the ideology surrounding their construction is bound up in the idea of the creation of a designated or bounded space for the accommodation and management of the insane. The maintenance of physical boundaries and the consolidation of spaces encouraged the creation and perpetuation of a dedicated institutional environment – both aesthetic and sensory. Within this institutional environment, the 'norms' of the asylum were established, allowing for the creation of delineating boundaries of 'order' and 'disorder'. The boundaries were policed by the staff as sentries, both physical and ideological, and the space was arranged to allow for their easy movement through it. This section has reconsidered the role of the 'unseen eye' and the panopticon, widely attributed to asylums in the secondary literature. Panoptic spaces, where they exist, may be seen as symbolic, embodying the architectural style of other institutions such as prisons and workhouses, but in practice requiring a more hands-on approach to the management of patients within. Ease of access and rapid response movement were a priority over remote surveillance.

The boundaries of the asylum were maintained by a focus on the creation of separate sensory spaces. This has been explored here in considering the control of the sensory environment through design innovation or the construction of separate spaces for the accommodation of 'noisy patients', convalescents, and everyone in between. This is articulated in the portrayal of the asylums in plans and in the didactic texts of the period, though in the documentary and material record it is difficult to locate sonic and visual experience.

Movement and access

The control and management of asylum spaces was central to the maintenance of the asylum as a self-contained and regulated institution. To create an environment of institutionalisation and impose order on the running of the building, careful control of access and movement was maintained. Control and management of interior and exterior spatial boundaries reinforced various hierarchical and occupational factors involved in the management of the asylum. In this final section, I will consider the hierarchy of access among staff and inmates at the asylum and determine the levels of access afforded to higher- and lower-level staff.

The privileges and levels of access granted to staff were varied. The asylum may be seen as an active space in constant flux, where internal boundaries were dictated by status of movement and hierarchies of access dependent on social position as attained through 'rites', such as admission and bathing for a patient (as discussed previously), or employment and promotion for staff. As noted by French anthropologist Arnold Van Gennep, the doorway or staircase may be seen as a boundary, which one must qualify by status to cross (1960: 25). Those spaces between – for example, hallways, waiting rooms, and parlours – may be considered liminal transitional spaces, where qualification took place and within which access could be challenged. The ground floor of the public asylum is the best example with which to illustrate these processes. In this section, access analysis maps demonstrate the points of access to the most prohibited asylum spaces: the individual patient rooms. The vestibule and entrance hall were spaces of scrutiny and qualification, enabling their occupants to pass through them into the next accessible stage.

Three access analysis maps (Figure 4.2) have been compiled for the Wakefield Asylum, the Richmond Lunatic Asylum, and the Irish provincial asylums, as general examples of the site type. They have been laid out in stages, so as best to demonstrate those areas which were roughly spatially related. Restricted spaces are located towards the extreme right of each map. The levels of access have been determined by joint consideration of the plans for each asylum (on construction) and the duties of staff detailed with regard to the asylums in the documentary record. The West Riding Asylum was constructed in such a manner as to allow for the dominance of the building's interior space by the manager and matron through their control of the central access staircases, which permitted access to upper floors. The wings were isolated and access to them was easily regulated by supervision of the corridors and the external exit on the northern wings of the ground floor. These external exits opened onto an enclosed courtyard; connected to the utilities block to the rear of the asylum, the yard space was enclosed by agents of supervision.

The Irish provincial asylums, represented here by Maryborough District Asylum, were constructed to allow for uninhibited movement through the asylum by the manager, housed in the central administration block. The manager's residence was both internally and externally similar to the Georgian architectural domestic styles favoured in the late eighteenth and early nineteenth centuries in nearby Dublin. The entrance to the residence was through a large internal door set into a

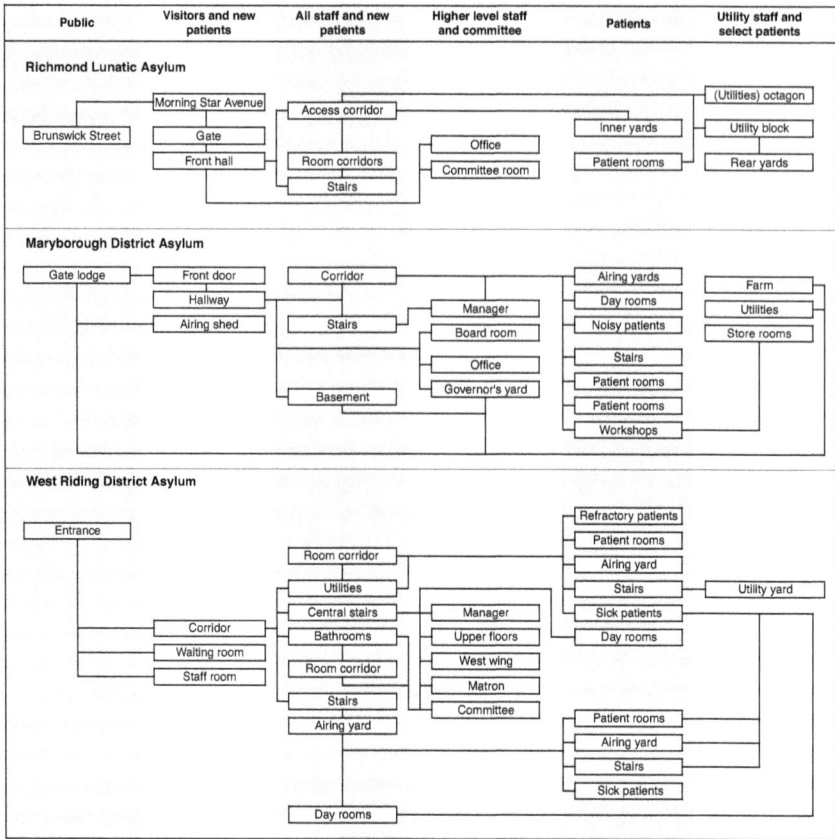

Figure 4.2 Access analyses of Richmond Lunatic Asylum, Maryborough District Asylum, and the West Riding District Asylum.

Georgian-style archway with glass panelling above the door, similar to upper-class terraced housing in Dublin's city centre. The residence allowed for the broadest unhindered access to several parts of the building, an access privilege not shared by any other area.

At Richmond Lunatic Asylum, the ground floor was served by a central access corridor, which allowed for access to the staircases leading to upper floors. The design of the building placed the patient rooms and access to the outside world in contraposition. The division of the floor into short nine-cell corridors suggests separation of inmates into small groups (of individuals, in patient rooms) as a primary means of maintaining order. Due to severe overcrowding in most asylums soon after they were constructed, careful division of small numbers of patients was made redundant quickly. In the Richmond Lunatic Asylum, as in many others of the period, overcrowding occurred as a result of unanticipated low numbers of discharges and the 'occupation of large numbers of incurables' (Copies of all Correspondence 1828).

In order to maintain control in the event of overcrowding, careful access to open corridors was practical. As with the Wakefield Asylum and the Maryborough District Asylum, external access at Richmond Lunatic Asylum was carefully controlled by a gate lodge and high walls. However, access to the asylum was further hindered by its construction within a built-up area, surrounded on three sides by other institutions (a workhouse, a surgical hospital, and a penitentiary) (Figure 4.3). The asylum, and access to it, was linked to access to other institutions, or at least geographical associations with them. Within the asylum, the highest levels of official access were afforded the manager and matron; though they would have had high-level access, free access to every room was not the privilege of general or support staff. In a letter outlining the duties of the staff of the Richmond District Lunatic Asylum in 1828, prior to the opening of the new asylum at Clonmel in the same year and in preparation for that, it was described that the moral manager was required to visit day rooms and maintain a familiarity with male patients, while female patients fell to the duty of the housekeeper and matron, who was also responsible for the maintenance of the entire house (Copies of all Correspondence 1828).

The duties of the matron, and her position as woman of the house, afforded her a higher level of access than the manager, despite the fact that he occupied the top position in the social hierarchy. In his highly critical account of the Wakefield Asylum, and notes on how it could be improved, Wakefield-based physician Caleb Crowther criticised the practice of awarding the position of matron to the wife of the manager. He stated that the duties of the matron should have been in attending each female patient every day and attending to the patient's comforts, as well as maintaining the house as housekeeper (Crowther 1838). This suggests that though her duties required her to be a housekeeper and to visit each female patient once a day, the matron at the Wakefield Asylum was at risk of compromising her position by her status as a woman with social interests and concerns.

Accounts of the duties of the matron indicate her role as requiring active contact with patients, keepers, and support staff in the utility blocks – more so than her male counterpart. Despite the duties expected and the power held by the matron in her access privileges, the matron was not in receipt of the same level of wages as the manager or even the visiting physician. By 1834, the matron at Richmond Lunatic Asylum was afforded a separate wage of £55.7.8 per annum, apart from her husband (the manager) whose wage totalled £250 per annum. At the

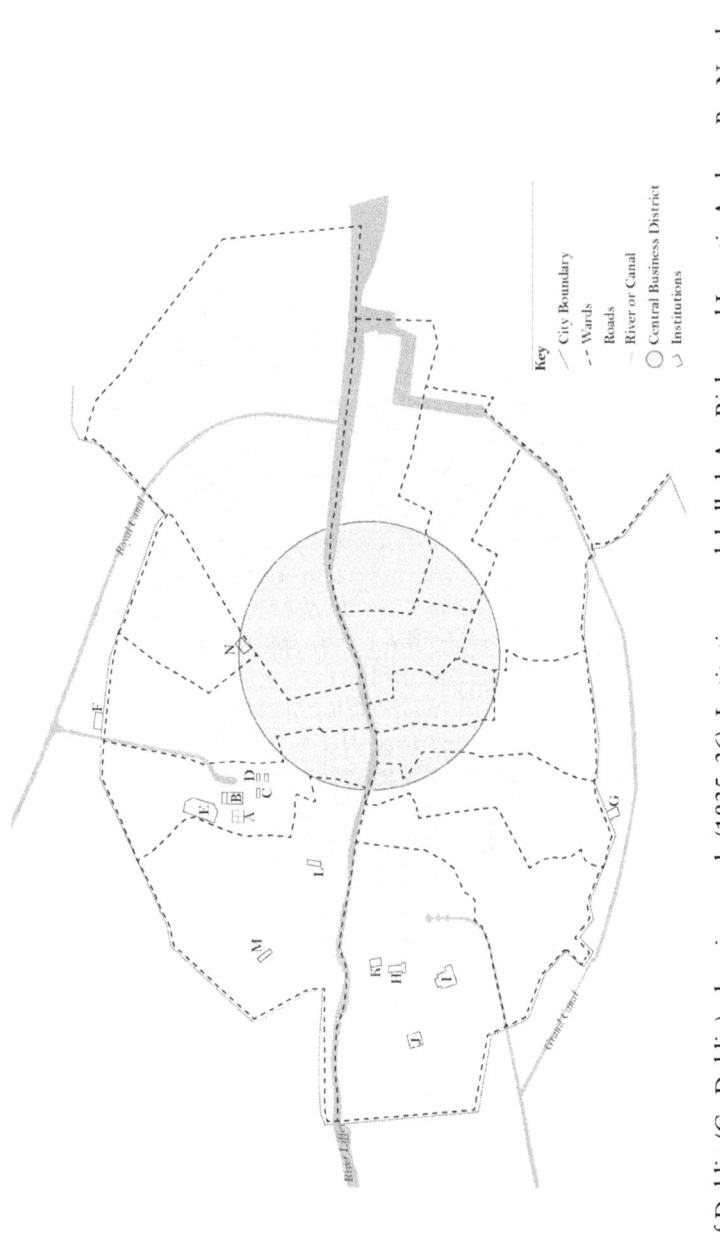

Figure 4.3 Plan of Dublin (Co Dublin), showing wards (1835–36). Institutions are labelled: A – Richmond Lunatic Asylum; B – North Dublin Union Workhouse and Bedford Asylum; C – Whitworth Hospital; D – Hardwick Hospital and Lunatic Asylum; E – Richmond Penitentiary; F – Female Penitentiary; G – Richmond Penitentiary; H – Swift's Hospital; I – South Dublin Union Workhouse; J – Royal Hospital; K – Steevens' Hospital; L – Bluecoat Hospital; M – Provost Hospital; N – Rotunda Hospital.

regional asylums, such as at the Maryborough District Asylum and Armagh District Asylum in the same period, the manager and matron received a joint wage of £250. It may be suggested that the position of the matron as head of in-house running was assumed, given her status as the wife of the manager (The National Archives of the United Kingdom Commissioners for Auditing: AO 2/68), reflecting domestic hierarchies in upper-class British and Irish Georgian households. This further supports the imposition of a domestic, rather than explicitly institutional, hierarchical regime within the asylum.

Within the asylum a hierarchy existed to operate within a specified social order, which was reinforced by the perpetuation and maintenance of roles delineated by space and access privilege. The asylum was carefully mapped to allow for the controlled and regulated access of certain people through certain spaces. However, human agency must be taken into account, and those boundaries and access points must be considered dynamic and subject to the control of those managing them. The internal hierarchy of the lunatic asylum, represented for example in a payroll, placed the manager at the top, followed by the matron, physician, clerk, and general and support staff: the keepers, attendants, laundry workers, and farm labourers (The National Archives of the United Kingdom Audits of Maryborough: AO 19/48/14; The National Archives of the United Kingdom Commissioners for Auditing: AO 2/68). This internal hierarchy was challenged with regard to the levels of access allowed for each staff member. The matron was the only staff member with unlimited access, both internally and externally, though officially the affairs of the asylum were represented and superintended by the manager. This hierarchical arrangement which placed the alpha female in charge of the running and maintenance of the house, with her husband as the primary administrator and named head, paralleled the contemporaneous late Georgian home hierarchies in upper-class houses. In this case, the matron was an acting 'mother' to patients, while the manager represented an austere and distant 'father' figure to whom everyone was ultimately answerable.

Boundaries and bound space

Building on earlier chapters on management and the maintenance of a bureaucracy, this chapter has focused on the application of those previously mentioned ideologies in the material operation of the asylum. The practicalities of movement and management in the lunatic asylum, as articulated through the control of space and the maintenance of strict boundaries, has been critically assessed with reference to architectural features and styles commonly ascribed to asylums. The asylum, in architectural terms, has often been equated to other contemporaneous institutions of the period, namely prisons and workhouses. The panopticon, for instance, is an architectural feature commonly attributed to all institutions for confinement in the early nineteenth century, including asylums. However, correspondence from the period, plans of contemporaneous asylums, and analysis of the spaces of these buildings suggest that the panopticon, as a fully functioning feature in the asylum, could not have been imposed on the purpose-built lunatic asylum due to conflict between the operation of a panoptic institution and the principles of moral management. The unpredictability and the broad and public nature of lunatic asylum accommodation could not allow for a catch-all surveillance or supervision system. Such a system could not facilitate the active management and care of patients. The presence of the keeper and the necessity for active supervision and physical presence was articulated in the construction of the bird nests in the Wakefield Asylum, and in the closed, self-contained corridors in Richmond Lunatic Asylum and provincial Irish asylums. However, the installation of panoptic-style features in the architecture of the asylum cannot be discounted: the construction of cupolas and features such as the octagonal towers suggest a role for the panoptic aesthetic in the asylum as a stylistic feature. Cupolas in particular created a focal point for viewing the asylum from the outside and reinforced the sense of order and classification in the asylum by emphasising the symmetry of the architecture and division into two gendered wings. This chapter demonstrates the degree to which specialised management of patients within the asylum, as well as the aesthetics of management, affected the institutional architecture imposed upon it by popular ideology and public expectation.

The cultivation of an interior sensory environment is worthy of further study. This chapter has outlined the concern for the sensory environment in didactic literature and asylum design. These concerns manifested themselves in the adoption of mortice locks to counter the noise of bolts and the use of low floors and high, rounded cills to enable light in patient rooms. As the Maryborough District Asylum is still standing with many original features, the building represents an opportunity to record the interior environment before the completion of hospital closure in favour of other styles of mental healthcare provision. Though there are difficulties associated with recording the interior sonic environment due to re-plastering of walls, double-glazing of windows, and division of corridors with fire doors, the remains of vaulted ceilings and stone floors could be examined to draw conclusions about the distribution of sound. How individuals and hierarchies operated within these dynamic spaces indicates that asylum spaces were more fluid and less proscribed than plans of the buildings suggest.

5

Conclusions

In the summer of 2016, the *Irish Times* newspaper published the text of a twenty-nine-page document discovered by an Irish student in the 1980s (Boland 2016). Penned by an anonymous former staff member of St Ita's Hospital outside Dublin, formerly Portrane Asylum, the document provided an account of daily life in the institution from the mid-twentieth century and a brief account of the history of the asylum. The document came to the student through a doctor, who pulled it from a filing cabinet as he showed the student around the building, and it formed the basis for that student's dissertation (Jones 1990). The attention provoked online by the article reflects the ongoing interest in historic asylums, while the publication of the account demonstrates an awareness of the importance of accounting for the history of these ever-changing and little-understood institutions. The main purpose of this book has been to present the dichotomy between the rhetoric of reform which surrounded asylum design, and operational practice in the first fifty years of the public asylum system. This was a period of significant change and innovation on the part of asylum designers and reformers, and asylums were not conceived of as standardised or static but were ever-changing and self-reflective. The impact of this period of experimentation can be seen in the decorative and domestic features which carried over into the Victorian asylums and which adorned the asylum at Enniscorthy causing such confusion locally.

Lunatic asylums were the proving grounds for architectural innovation and idealism. Their design and management significantly influenced a new generation of asylums based on the revision of their Georgian predecessors in the second half of the nineteenth and into the twentieth century. The 1845 Lunacy Acts initiated a new hierarchy of responsibility based on regular inspection and strict bureaucracy (Taylor 1995: 15). These new asylums were informed by physicians like John Conolly (1847), whose treatise on the characteristics of ideal lunatic asylum design has placed him at the forefront of writing on asylum architecture

(Edington 2007: 85; Hine 1901; Piddock 2007, 2009; Taylor 1991; Thompson and Goldin 1975). Victorian asylum architects drew on architectural influences beyond the standard neo-classical style which defined their Georgian predecessors: innovations in management style and corridor layout, as well as material features such as reinforced windows. As such, by the end of the nineteenth century, asylum architecture became more consolidated, bearing less resemblance to the country-house style of institutions like the York Retreat than to general hospitals and other asylums.

Moral management, though occupying a significant position in the establishment of a lunatic asylum system, was in early practice nuanced and specific in application to individual institutions. Similarly, the design principles which informed the development of asylum architecture were site specific and bound closely to the financial means of those who were overseeing construction. The choice of lunatic asylum design was significantly influenced by both monetary concerns and the maintenance of a moral character in the institution. Designs such as the panopticon, which were expensive and geared towards confinement and control, were wholly unsuitable, particularly in light of the concerns of men like Samuel Tuke for whom designing a purpose-built asylum separate in character and practice from prisons was paramount. Lunatic asylum architecture had more in common with country-house architecture in terms of landscaping, domestic interior design, and security. This is evidenced by the provision of expansive gardens and plantations, interior spatial and material layout, and the inclusion of features such as gate lodges. In their determination to implement a domestic environment, asylum reform theorists like Tuke, Charlesworth, and Conolly were concerned with delineating the management of lunatic asylums as social institutions separate in nature and mission from prisons, houses of industry, and even general infirmaries. These concerns can be clearly seen as articulated in the material remains of the institution and supported in the documentary source material. Crucially, from a methodological perspective, material culture and material traces in the documentary record can be utilised in order to determine everyday practice. The strength of the method employed here is the collaborative use of material remains and historical documents. Documentary sources both locate and situate material remains where none survive today. The material, both documentary and artefactual, gained from this approach offers an insight into everyday practice. The sources and material presented in this book address the progress and practice of reform in different spheres of asylum life, all of which are visible in the material and documentary record.

Management practice was reviewed in terms of how practice related to the ideals espoused in the didactic literature of the period. The extent to which each individual manager was capable of implementing moral management in their respective asylums was limited by the expertise and quality of lower-level staff and the demands of the public. Management practice was further constrained by the limitations and boundaries of the space of the asylums. Asylum architecture has been presented as a specialist genre, in common yet separate from other contemporaneous institutions like prisons and workhouses. While surveillance was a concern, this concern was not addressed through the use of simplistic spatial organisation according to principles such as Bentham's panopticon. In place of an all-seeing eye from which the patients could be watched, surveillance was carried out through active movement and sensory engagement with the material space of the buildings. The sensory environment was thus central to the experience of the space of the actors within and was a concern for reformers during the design process. Negotiation of asylum space was contingent on priority or privilege of access. A comparison of asylum plans and the documentary records led to the conclusion that the highest privilege of access in the asylum, through duties and position, was afforded to the matron. The matron is a somewhat shadowy figure in the critical literature on asylums, despite the fact that she was afforded the greatest degree of familiarity with patients and staff on an everyday basis, and her duties meant that she was expected to know the asylum – patients, staff, and building – thoroughly. Though the asylum hierarchy was designed along the patriarchal lines of domestic dwellings, the duties of the matron meant that she was a more frequently encountered authority figure than the manager in the practical running of the institution.

As much of the historical record was composed of bureaucratic materials, such as accounts and reports, it is not surprising that the manager was more commonly represented than any other staff member. It has been possible to draw conclusions based on official quarterly or annual reports. The large amount of source material encountered in the course of this research raised questions about where and how that material was managed and stored and who interacted with it. The process of admission has been singled out as a bureaucratic process involving a large number of actors, from the gatekeeper to the patient, and was an essential ritual in the running of the asylum. Asylum designers were heavily influenced by country-house architecture, and the rituals undertaken in the admission process – while akin to those undertaken at workhouses – were also bound up in the hierarchy of the middle-class domestic home. This was reflected in the paternalistic relationship between the state and the asylum.

The conclusions reached through this analysis of the built

environment and material management of asylums contribute to the scholarship on the historical archaeology of institutions and lunatic asylum archaeology by assessing the practical application of the rhetoric of reform and considering the roles of staff members who fall outside official narratives and more traditional histories of medicine. The early nineteenth-century asylum is presented here as a dynamic archaeological space whose material environment was constantly changed on reflection and revisions in thinking about mental health. The artefact-based approach to reading and handling the documentary sources employed in this book establishes the value in populating the historical record with material culture and supplementing the material record with documents generated through institutional bureaucracy. In turn, this approach has contributed to the existing literature on patient and staff experience by showing how material culture, specifically the materials of bureaucracy (i.e. paper and books) and the architecture itself, influenced the way spaces were arranged and negotiated by actors on a daily basis. As such, the built heritage of the asylum extends beyond the shell of the buildings themselves. Both the asylum interiors and the landscapes which surround them must be seen as part of asylum heritage. Landscapes and interiors frequently fall outside considerations of the built heritage of asylum. Both features of the asylum which reflect therapeutic aspects of moral management, their omission from consideration leaves the sometimes austere-looking asylum buildings themselves to speak for the legacy of their institutions. The ways in which these buildings are approached by developers, the public, and even scholars reflect public discomfort with these institutions that persists into the present day.

Heritage and the legacy of *asylumdom*

The material remains of the lunatic asylum system have captured the popular imagination as the dark and (sometimes) decaying facades of former asylums offer suitable backdrops to a collective discomfort with the idea of mental illness and the treatment methods that developed in asylums from the late eighteenth century. In the introduction to this book, I mentioned the use of lunatic asylums as rich settings for fictional horror and violence, citing as an example the Danvers State Asylum in Massachusetts, H.P. Lovecraft's inspiration for his Arkham Sanitarium. The Arkham Sanitarium's more famous namesake, Arkham Asylum, from the DC Comics *Batman* series, is an even more explicit showcase of gothic horror, represented architecturally with Victorian elements in comics, films, and video games and playing host to the most notorious villains of Gotham City. This correlation between criminality and mental illness is not uncommon in popular representations of lunatic asylums.

It is this correlation, however, which has a potentially damaging impact on how real asylum buildings are treated after they cease to be used as hospitals. The representation of architecture in print and digital media, and particularly in an immersive experience like a video game, can have an effect on the observers' or players' perception of the buildings and environments in reality (Dow 2013: 223). If a fictional asylum is represented as a place of dark heritage, a real asylum may be seen in the same light. The view of asylums as places of dark history is compounded by their own built heritage, which is frequently dark in a physical sense.

In his analysis of early nineteenth-century Irish asylum architecture, Markus Reuber described boarded-up lunatic asylums as a common sight on the outskirts of Irish towns (1996: 1179). The unlit, uncleaned, stone edifices of disused lunatic asylums were a common sight in England and Ireland during the 1990s, when Reuber was carrying out his research. Even before they were vacated, the utility of the imposing architecture of the buildings was a talking point, as the purposes to which they could be put were as much in question as the services which could reasonably be provided in them as working hospitals.

> There they stand, isolated, majestic, imperious, brooded over by the gigantic water-tower and chimney combined, rising unmistakable and daunting out of the countryside – the asylums which our forefathers built with such immense solidity to express the notions of their day. (Powell 1961)

Enoch Powell's impassioned speech as British Minister of Health in 1961 neatly sums up mid-twentieth-century frustration with the Georgian and Victorian buildings that made up the bulk of the country's mental healthcare facilities. Rebuilding in bombed-out cities, economic upturn, and the establishment of new government bodies like the National Health Service in the wake of the Second World War saw the proliferation of modernist architecture and the material realisation of new ideas about urban planning and civic infrastructure across the British Isles. The building boom placed the Georgian and Victorian architecture, which formed the core of many asylums, in a new light. These buildings were no longer deemed suitable for the purpose for which they were constructed. In addition, improvements in the treatment of mental illness were inspiring legislative change, moving away from the idea of the asylum and towards community care. In his 'Water Tower' speech, Powell was speaking at the Annual Conference of the National Association for Mental Health, in his first year of office and in the wake of the 1959 Mental Health Act (7 & 8. Eliz.2, c. 72), which introduced the goal of community care and removed the distinction between mental hospitals and other hospitals. The Act is significant in the history of mental healthcare as it legislated for the eventual abolition of an institutional solution to the treatment of the mentally ill. As such, it was incumbent on the new Minister of Health to reinforce the idea that mental hospitals, many occupying Georgian and Victorian buildings, were not fit for long-term purpose. It is significant that Powell was also a cabinet member in Harold Macmillan's Conservative government which was at the time overseeing massive slum clearance projects and the construction of new towns organised along modernist principles.

Powell's choice of words in his 'Water Tower' speech presents asylums as impressive carry-overs from a bygone age of architectural prowess. He further points out that, by 1961, they were innocuous in the British landscape. The number of asylums, this suggests, somewhat dilutes their impressiveness. The water tower and chimney of the large Victorian asylum were no doubt familiar sights to the denizens of city and countryside alike, particularly in the area around London where massive asylum buildings from the mid-nineteenth century, like the Second Middlesex Asylum at Colney Hatch, were still in operation. Powell counters any would-be objectors to the destruction of the Georgian and Victorian asylums, arguing that the buildings were never built to last, and juxtaposing the increasingly weatherworn lunatic asylums with famous sites of archaeological significance, specifically the Pyramids of Giza. 'Hospital building is not like pyramid building', he stated, 'the erection of memorials to endure to a remote posterity' (1961). Rather, he suggested that hospital buildings should be seen as a physical framework in which to facilitate treatment. The ideals of men like Tuke and Charlesworth, to create therapeutic landscapes beyond the shells of the buildings themselves, had clearly not been borne out, given that men in positions like Powell's could not see the asylum site as holistic, focusing on the buildings. Asylums were no longer useful, he implied, so their destruction was necessary. No stranger to inflammatory, evocative language, as the controversy surrounding his later and more famous 'Rivers of Blood' speech indicates, Powell used imagery in his 'Water Tower' speech to communicate the failings and inadequacies of a mental healthcare system that was undergoing yet another period of significant change. He went on to advocate for the introduction of a community-based system of care according to the latest proposals for reform in mental health treatment. Significantly, the adoption of community care would mean a reduction of the extent of institutional provision for the mentally ill, from large mental hospitals into purpose-built wards in general hospitals. Powell's words heralded a period of transformation and change in the management of mental health in Britain. Mental hospitals began to close their doors in the final decades of the twentieth century, leaving many former Georgian and Victorian asylum buildings empty, open for redevelopment, and in a few cases allowed to slump into dilapidation.

In Ireland, mental hospitals downsized at a slower rate, as the local mental hospital was explicitly tied to provincial employment and the rural economy (Brennan 2014: 119). The 1945 Mental Treatment Act laid the groundwork for the introduction of mental healthcare outside of the asylum, allowing for outpatient treatment. There were concerns regarding the institutional treatment of mental illness in the middle of the twentieth century and the stigma surrounding mental health; a Grangegorman Mental Hospital Board member complained in 1950, for example, that he had heard patients of that institution (the former Richmond Lunatic Asylum) referred to at a meeting of Dublin County Council as 'inmates' (Reynolds 1992: 281). Various government enquiries and reports followed the 1945 Mental Treatment Act advocating for a change in institutional provision for the mentally ill, most notably the Department of Health report *The Psychiatric Services – Planning for the Future* (1984). The adoption of community care in the second half of the twentieth century led to a downsizing of mental hospitals, and the 2001 Mental Health Act, which superseded the 1945 Act, provided for large-scale closure at last. Reuber's observation of boarded-up hospital buildings on town outskirts in 1996 captures the long, slow process of closure at work in Ireland since the 1980s; the 2001 Act only made the process official. By the 2010s new psychiatric units in general hospitals were taking new and short-term admissions. Patient numbers in the mental hospitals that remained open dwindled to the point that former asylum buildings were beginning to look empty. In 2010, the intention to sell former psychiatric hospitals and land was announced by the Minister of State (Prior 2012). The sale of the buildings and land would, it was envisioned, release equity to fund a new system for mental healthcare in Ireland (Government of Ireland 2006: 183). The government's advisory report, *A Vision for Change*, specifically noted the importance of developing a new system in buildings not affected by the stigma of historical institutionalisation (2006: 179). The disposal of the built heritage of the historical asylum was written into plans for moving forward, implying that the sites of past failures were too tied to those failures or inadequacies to play any part in a new system. The buildings themselves came to represent the outdated system of institutional confinement which had dominated mainstream approaches to mental health for two hundred years since the 1808 County Asylums Act.

In consequence of these legislative provisions for the closure of mental hospitals across the British Isles, many former asylum buildings stood empty, awaiting redevelopment. The spaces were infiltrated by those who had stood outside the system, without any connection to mental healthcare or treatment, notably artists who were keen to explore sites of popular myth. In the popular imagination, the abandoned historic lunatic asylum occupies an atmospheric niche between fear and anger. Urban explorers and photographers have explored the remains of former asylums, and evocative images of disused corridors strewn with medical equipment, beds, and myriad other debris of daily life have been published in photographic collections. A notable example is Christopher Payne's work in the book *Asylum*, which documents state mental hospitals in the United States (Payne and Sacks 2009). In light of such a reputation, and given popular associations with the buildings' histories, the repurposing of former asylum buildings in England and Ireland has been a slow process. Hazardous materials like asbestos on newer parts of the buildings and dilapidation due to neglect or asset stripping have compounded the problem of reputation and contributed to the reluctance of would-be developers, though the active ruination of the buildings has created more atmospheric spaces for photographers to capture. The dilapidation of closed asylums contributes to the negative reputation of the buildings and has impacted their candidacy for redevelopment – as the case of the Wakefield Asylum clearly demonstrates.

The core buildings of the Wakefield Asylum, like many former asylum buildings, have been redeveloped for residential use. Significantly for the redevelopment of the site, the building was listed in 1989 as Grade II ('of special interest, warranting every effort to preserve them'; Department of Culture, Media and Sport 2010: 4), with the original H-plan of the 1810s building cited as the most important architectural feature on the site. The listing for the Wakefield Asylum states the importance of the original building in influencing the architectural style of asylums, and notes that the building was heavily modified in the late nineteenth and early twentieth centuries. Critically, the listing only covers the eastern part of the asylum, the theatre, and Watson and Pritchett's ventilation shaft to the rear of the building. As such, when the building was converted to residential apartments in the early 2000s, the western end of the asylum, which had been constructed in the mid-to-late nineteenth and early twentieth centuries, was demolished. Interestingly, while the Georgian period of lunatic asylum development is largely passed over in favour of the Victorian asylums in the historiography and in the popular imagination, architecturally the earlier formative period is more likely to have survived due to pioneering architectural design and greater antiquity. The West Riding Asylum at Wakefield was, at the time of its closure at the end of the twentieth century, known as Stanley Royd Hospital. Unsurprisingly, neither the name of the asylum nor the later hospital survives in the modern development, which has been named Parklands Manor. In common with other former asylum sites, the names of doctors have been preserved in the surrounding residential streets (Tuke Grove, Bevan Grove, Ashworth Square), but the name of the site has been stripped from it. This is prevalent in former asylum buildings; the early Victorian Exe Vale Asylum was marketed as Devington Park by its developers, who argued that the majority of people would not like to live in a former mental hospital (Franklin 2002a: 177). In the absence of their name and identifying markers, 'the casual observer could be forgiven for mistaking a recycled asylum for the buildings and grounds of a refurbished stately home' (Joseph *et al.* 2013: 140). The impact of this identity stripping on the historical communities which grew up around asylums and hospitals remains to be seen.

As mental hospitals have closed, some buildings have not been reused or have been left for a long time without development. The resulting dilapidation and ruination of these large, now-purposeless buildings, has attracted a different kind of attention. Ruined asylum buildings have been vandalised and, in a few cases, destroyed. As the population of former patients and nurses who settled around asylums dwindles and communities break up, there is a far smaller population of invested individuals living around the buildings to ensure their preservation from harm. The sprawling mass of the early Victorian asylum, Our Lady's Hospital in Cork, Ireland was destroyed by fire in 2017, after lying empty for nearly a decade. Among the most vocal mourners of the building were the urban explorers for whom the asylum was popular. The distress of urban explorers and photographers attests to the graduation of the historic lunatic asylum from a marginal and unknown institution into a host for artistic expression. In addition to documenting the active ruination of former asylum buildings, urban explorers give a creative voice to public discomfort with institutional spaces. Through their art, a once-excluded general public can access asylum buildings, at once a domineering presence in the urban and rural landscape and a closed 'other' space about which those not actively employed or hospitalised know little. The photographs of urban explorers are widely engaged with, published and unpublished, adding a new historical layer to the asylums they engage with: a post-institutional phase. In documenting the surviving remains, urban explorers also document the abandonment and post-settlement phase (in archaeological terminology) of the asylum sites.

While commercial archaeologists document asylum buildings before demolition and redevelopment, recording the buildings before they cease being asylums or mental hospitals and become something else, their record of the buildings is frequently and necessarily focused on architectural features of particular interest. A standing building survey records the built heritage of the asylum in a manner that is useful to researchers and planners, but their job is not to communicate any sense of the asylum as an historical place. Though problematic in their means of acquiring subject material, and sometimes hyperbolic or salacious in their expression, urban explorers are concerned with identifying and capturing aspects of the building's heritage which communicate the building's use as a hospital in a subjective and historically aware manner. As such, the emotional history of the buildings is recorded in a manner not usually open to commercial archaeologists and frequently overlooked by researchers. A collaboration between the interested communities associated with buildings like asylums – in this case urban explorers – and those concerned with preserving the sites (even if only in plan or photograph) would open up dialogue about the later history of the sites after closure and aid in preserving emotional ties. As this book has argued, the historic asylum building was an active landscape and taskscape, where the personal geographies and concerns of individual agents frequently impacted the layout or use of different parts of the buildings. While this aspect of the built heritage is difficult to pin down empirically, it is nevertheless an aspect of the building's history and an aspect of the intangible heritage of asylums. The emotional history and archaeology of lunatic asylums is intrinsic to the way the buildings are interacted with by the public, by developers, by researchers, and by artists. As such, the visual interpretation of such spaces should be taken into account in the management and planning for such buildings.

Returning to the idea of the asylum as a site of dark heritage, the encounters between the public and former asylum buildings themselves suggest that the lunatic asylum is considered a site of dark and difficult history. However, not every engagement with the sites in their 200-year history has been negative, and their foundation was not attended with an idea of prolonged human suffering in mind. Lunatic asylums had no singular purpose to pin a very dark history too, but they are undoubtedly sites of difficult emotional history. According to Philip Stone's typology of dark tourism sites (2006: 151), lunatic asylums stand somewhere in the middle of the spectrum, occupying a dark-grey space between the darkest heritage and the lighter shades of difficult histories: they were constructed for long timescales and huge, diverse populations; they have been maintained for first practical and then conservation purposes; and the histories of these spaces have been occluded and curated by different groups. Historically, materially, and emotionally, lunatic asylum sites are more nuanced than they have been perceived.

Concluding thoughts

This book calls for the consideration of lunatic asylums as distinct institutions separate in ethos and architectural rhetoric to prisons and workhouses. The centrality of the asylum buildings to historical communities who grew up around them show that they were not problematically peripheral or marginal (or 'dark') to those who interacted with them on a daily basis, which included communities of staff and patients that sometimes numbered into the high hundreds. This book argues that asylum buildings are themselves victims of their own essential nature to the communities they were constructed in. Though many asylum architects were concerned with the creation of specialist asylum buildings for use by people with needs beyond incarceration or punishment, they were constrained by budget and materials. Despite noble intentions, the early ideology within which much of the didactic literature and asylum plans were composed was fundamentally flawed, presupposing that madness was homogenous and curable in a period before pharmacology. Demographic and economic demand, as well as the activities of individual actors within the buildings, were culpable in breaking apart this ideology. The overcrowding and overuse of early nineteenth-century asylums led directly to major redesign, and a reassessment of architecture and management practice in the asylums built after 1845.

The buildings at the centre of this research, Georgian lunatic asylums, currently enjoy Grade II listed or protected status in England and Ireland. This book has endeavoured to illustrate the importance of the interior environment and the surrounding grounds to the buildings as a whole in the planning of the buildings for reform and in their practical operation. Focus is drawn from the basic outline of the building, which is generally the only aspect of the original design remaining following redevelopment. Retention of the shell of the main buildings promotes the 'stately home' aspect of the design when they are converted to residences (Franklin 2002b: 29–31), and also sidesteps the problems and stigma associated with the more clinical – 'darker' – aspects of the interior. The moral rhetoric and innovative approaches to the architecture of Georgian asylums informed the interior, as well as exterior, of the buildings. This is important to consider in the redevelopment of institutional sites; though the historical record generally maintains plans and records for buildings, the internal fabric can be indicative of lived environment, staff and patient experience, and negotiation of space. As such, the interior as well as exterior designs should be considered in the architectural appraisal of these buildings while they are still recognisable as hospitals. Asylum architecture must be considered as a whole, interior and exterior, in order to understand the intentions and issues associated with management practice.

By focusing on lunatic asylums as workplaces, hospitals, care-orientated buildings, and institutions of social and mental improvement, this outlook has implications for the redevelopment of lunatic asylum sites and the popular understanding of these buildings which has impacted their reuse. The popular cultural memory of lunatic asylums as places of incarceration, abuse, and control is articulated in literature and film. Popular representations of lunatic asylums as coercive and inhumane contribute to the marginalisation of these buildings on a local level. In turn, this marginalisation has led to the destruction or rebranding of redeveloped institutions, effectively removing any association with mental illness from the communities that once grew up around them. Small communities who then become responsible for the asylum's material culture in museums and private collections do not want the memory of the institution as a community focus to be lost. The centrality of the asylum to its local community – both in the past and today – is evidenced in the proliferation of community run museums, in the interest of urban exploration groups and artists, and in historical accounts like that mentioned at the start of this chapter. The continued problematic treatment of these spaces as marginal, difficult, and 'scary' implies a level of social stigma regarding mental illness that is contrary to drives towards its social acceptance in the twenty-first century and initiatives spearheaded by mental health charities and government bodies. The deserted corridors and half-furnished remains of many former asylums in the British Isles offer an evocative canvas on which the history of mental health may be imposed, but this may obscure the lived histories of these buildings. Closer examination of the ideas and rhetoric behind the construction of these buildings, some striking enough to make convincing apartment buildings and hotels, should inform this narrative so that stigma and fear of mental illness do not mar the legacy of these buildings and the history of their associated communities of staff and patients.

References

Abbott, William. (1833a). Advertisement for Gardener. *The Leinster Express*, 20 April 1833.
__ (1833b). Announcement of Opening. *The Leinster Express*, 4 May 1833.
Akehurst, A. (2010). The York Retreat. A vernacular of equality. In: Guillery, P. (ed.). *Built from Below: British Architecture and the Vernacular*. London: Routledge.
Alborn, Timothy. (2010). Economics and business. In: Gorman, Francis (ed.) *The Cambridge Companion to Victorian Culture*. Cambridge: Cambridge University Press.
Anderson, Gregory. (1976). *Victorian Clerks*. Manchester: Manchester University Press.
Andrews, J., A. Briggs, R. Porter, P. Tucker, and K. Waddington. (1997). *The History of Bethlem*. London: Routledge.
Anonymous. (1839). District Lunatic Asylums. *Dublin Medical Press* 1(21).
__ (1902). The annual museum of foods, drugs, instruments, books and sanitary appliances. *The British Medical Journal* 2(2172): 459–466.
A Return of the Number of Houses in Each County, or Division of the County, Licensed for the Reception of Lunatics the Names of the Persons to whom the Licences are Granted; as well as the Number of Patients Confined in Each House; Distinguishing Males and Females; 1819 (271).
Arnold, Catharine. (2008). *Bedlam: London and Madness*. London: Simon & Schuster.
Ashworth, A.L. (1975). *Stanley Royd Hospital, Wakefield: One Hundred and Fifty Years. A History*. Wakefield: Stanley Royd Hospital.
Augst, Thomas. (2003). *The Clerk's Tale*. London: University of Chicago Press.
Baines, Edward. (1822). *History, Directory and Gazetteer of the County of York, with select lists of merchants and traders of London and the principal commercial and manufacturing Towns of England; and a variety of other commercial information: also a copious list of the Seats of the Nobility and Gentry of Yorkshire*. Leeds: Edward Baines.
Bartlett, Peter. (1998). The asylum, the workhouse, and the voice of the insane poor in 19th-century England. *International Journal of Law and Psychiatry* 21(4): 421–432.
Battie, William. (1758). *A Treatise on Madness*. London: Whiston and White.
Beck, Tony. (2011). Charles Smith & Sons Ltd, Birmingham – Lock Manufacturers,

Bellhangers, Brass Founders & Whitesmiths: from 1828 to c. 1940. *The Lock Collector* (30): 7–10.
Bentham, Jeremy. (1791). *Panopticon: Postscript; Part I containing further particulars and alterations relative to the Plans of Construction originally posed; Principally adopted to the Purpose of a Panopticon Penitentiary House.* London: T. Payne.
Bethlem Royal Hospital Archives: Maps and plans of land and buildings on the hospital site at St George's Fields, Southwark 1837–1852.
Bewley, Thomas. (2008). *Madness to Mental Illness: A History of the Royal College of Psychiatrists*. London: RCPsych Publications.
Bhabha, Homi K. (1994). *The Location of Culture*. London: New York: Routledge.
Bigelow, Gordon. (2003). *Fiction, Famine and the Rise of Economics in Victorian Britain and Ireland*. Cambridge: Cambridge University Press.
Blesser, Barry and Salter, Linda Ruth. (2007). *Spaces Speak, Are You Listening? Experiencing Aural Architecture*. Cambridge: MIT Press.
Boland, Rosita. (2016). 'Isolated from the Mainstream': Portrane Asylum in the 1950s. *The Irish Times,* 10 June 2016.
Bolton, Joseph Shaw. (1928). The evolution of a mental hospital. *Journal of Medical Science* 74: 588–633.
Boyd, Gary. (2006). *Dublin, 1745–1922: Hospitals, Spectacle and Vice*. Dublin: Four Courts Press.
Brennan, Damien. (2014). *Irish Insanity: 1800–2000*. London: Routledge.
Briggs, Asa. (2000). *The Age of Improvement, 1783–1867*. 2nd edn. Harlow: Pearson Education Limited.
Brown, Pat. (2008). Fundamentals of Audio and Acoustics. In: Ballou, Glen M. (ed.) *Handbook for Sound Engineers*. 4th edn. Oxford: Focal.
Brown, Richard. (2003). *Church and State in Modern Britain 1700–1850*. London: Routledge.
Browne, W.A.F. (1991). What asylums were, are and ought to be. In: Scull, Andrew T. (ed.) *The Asylum as Utopia: W.A.F. Browne and the Mid-Nineteenth Century Consolidation of Psychiatry*. London: Routledge.
Burdett, Henry C. (1891). *Hospitals and Asylums of the World*. London: J. & A. Churchill.
Burke, John. (1832). *A General and Heraldic Dictionary of the Peerage and Baronetage of the British Empire*. 4th edn. London: Henry Coleburn and Richard Bently.
Burman, Barbara (2003). Pocketing the difference: Gender and pockets in nineteenth century Britain. In: Burman, Barbara and Turbin, Carole (eds). *Material Strategies: Dress and Gender in Historical Perspective*. Oxford: Blackwell.
Busetto, Giorgio. (2008). *Small Collection of Antique Silver and Objects of Vertu* [Online]. Venice. Available: www.silvercollection.it/electroplatesilverKLdue.html [Accessed 4 May 2012].
Butler, R.M. (2015). The reconstruction of O'Connell Street, Dublin. *Studies: An Irish Quarterly Review* 5(20): 570–576.
Campbell Clark, A., McIvor Campbell, C., and Turnbull, A.R. (1885). *Handbook for Attendants on the Insane*. London: Bailliere.
Carpenter, Diane. (2010). Above all a patient should never be terrified: an examina-

tion of mental health care and treatment in Hampshire 1845–1914. PhD Thesis, University of Plymouth.

Casella, Eleanor Conlin. (2002). *Archaeology of the Ross Female Factory: Female Incarceration in Van Diemen's Land, Australia (Records of the Queen Victoria Museum Volume 108)*. Launceston: Queen Victoria Museum & Art Gallery.

__ (2005). Prisoner of His Majesty: postcoloniality and the archaeology of British penal transportation. *World Archaeology* 37(3): 453–467.

__ (2007). *The Archaeology of Institutional Confinement*. Gainesville: University Press of Florida.

__ (2009). Written on the walls: Inmate graffiti within places of confinement. In: Beisaw, April M. and Gibb, James G. (eds). *The Archaeology of Institutional Life*. Tuscaloosa: The University of Alabama Press.

Casey, Christine and Rowan, Alexander. (1993). *Buildings of Ireland: North Leinster*. London: Penguin.

Charlesworth, E.P. (1828). *Remarks on the Treatment of the Insane: And the Management of Lunatic Asylums*. London: Rivington.

Chief Secretary's Office Registered Papers. (1821). Letter from Dr Francis Leigh, Dublin, requesting employment as medical superintendent of asylum. National Archives of Ireland CSO/RP/1821/1784.

Christie, Christopher. (2000). *The British Country Houses in the Eighteenth Century*. Manchester: Manchester University Press.

Cocroft, Wayne and Wilson, Louise K. (2006). Archaeology and art at Spadeadam Rocket Establishment (Cumbria). In: Schofield, John, Klausmeier, Axel, and Purbrick, Louise (eds). *Re-mapping the Field: New Approaches in Conflict Archaeology*. Bonn: Westkreuz-Verlag.

Coleborne, Catharine. (2010). *Madness in the Family: Insanity and Institutions in the Australasian Colonial World, 1860–1914*. Basingstoke: Palgrave Macmillan.

Conolly, J. (1847). *The Construction and Government of Lunatic Asylums and Hospitals for the Insane*. London: John Churchill.

__ (1856). *The Treatment of the Insane Without Mechanical Restraints*. London: Smith, Elder, and Co.

Copies of all Correspondence and Communications between the Home Office and the Irish Government, during the year 1827, on the Subject of Public Lunatic Asylums; 1828 (234).

Cooper, T. (2008). Archaeological desk-based assessment at Crooked Acres, Kirkstall, Leeds. ARCUS Report No. 11671.1.

Corbin, Alain. (1995). *Time, Desire and Horror: Towards a History of the Senses*. Cambridge: Polity Press.

__ (2004). Identity, bells, and the nineteenth-century French village. In: Smith, Mark M. (ed.) *Hearing History: a Reader*. London: The University of Georgia Press.

Corsellis, C.C. (1832). The Thirteenth Report of the Director of the West-Riding of York Pauper Lunatic Asylum. *County Lunatic Asylum Reports*. Wakefield: R. Hurst.

__ (1833). The Fourteenth Report of the Director of the West-Riding of York Pauper Lunatic Asylum. *County Lunatic Asylum Reports*. Wakefield: R. Hurst.

__ (1842). The Twenty-Third Report of the Director of the West-Riding of York Pauper Lunatic Asylum. *County Lunatic Asylum Reports*. Wakefield: R. Hurst.

__ (1844). The Twenty-Fifth Report of the Director of the West-Riding of York

Pauper Lunatic Asylum. *County Lunatic Asylums Report*. Wakefield: R. Hurst.
County Council of Surrey. (1929). *Rules for the Guidance of the Nurses, Attendants, & Servants in the Service of the Surrey County Mental Hospitals at Brookwood and Netherne*. Brookwood: Council of Surrey.
Craig, Maurice. (1982). *The Architecture of Ireland from the Earliest Times to 1880*. London: B.T. Batsford Ltd.
Cross, K.W., Harrington, J.A., and Mayer-Gross, W. (1957). A survey of chronic patients in a mental hospital. *The British Journal of Psychiatry* 103: 146–171.
Cross, S. (2012). Bedlam in mind: Seeing and reading historical images of madness. *European Journal of Cultural Studies* 15(1): 19–34.
Crossman, Virginia. (2006). *The Poor Law in Ireland 1838–1948*. Studies in Irish Economic and Society History Volume 10. Dublin: Dundalk.
Crossrail. (2017). 'The New Churchyard.' *Crossrail Archaeology* [Online]. Available: http://archaeology.crossrail.co.uk/ [Accessed 13 December 2017].
Crowther, Caleb. (1838). *Observations on the Management of Madhouses, Illustrated by Occurrences in the West Riding and Middlesex Asylums*. London: Simpkin, Marshall, and Co.
Curl, James Stevens and Wilson, Susan. (2015). *The Oxford Dictionary of Architecture 3rd Edition*. Oxford: Oxford University Press.
Davies, John E. (1994). Giffen goods, the survival imperative, and the Irish potato culture. *Journal of Political Economy* 102(3): 547–565.
De Cunzo, Lu Ann. (2001). On reforming the 'fallen' and beyond: Transforming continuity at the Magdalen Society of Philadelphia, 1845–1916. *International Journal of Historical Archaeology* 5(1): 19–43.
__ (2006). Exploring the institution: Reform, confinement, social change. In: Hall, Martin and Silliman, Stephen W. (eds). *Historical Archaeology*. Oxford: Blackwell Publishing.
Delle, James A. (1998). *An Archaeology of Social Space: Analyzing Coffee Plantations in Jamaica's Blue Mountains*. London: Plenum Press.
Department of Culture, Media and Sport. (2010). *Principles of Selection for Listing Buildings*. Gov.uk Guidance Document.
Department of Health. (1984). *The Psychiatric Services – Planning for the Future*. Dublin: The Stationery Office.
Dickens, Charles. (1861). *Great Expectations*. Leipzig: Bernhard Tauchnitz.
Dow, Douglas N. (2013). Historical veneers: anachronism, simulation, and art history in *Assassin's Creed II*. In: Kappell, Matthew Wilhelm and Elliot, Andrew B.R. (eds). *Playing with the Past: Digital Games and the Simulation of History*. London: Bloomsbury Academic.
Driver, Felix. (2004). *Power and Pauperism: The Workhouse System, 1834–1884*. Cambridge: Cambridge University Press.
Dunning, Phil. (2000). Composite table cutlery from 1700–1930. In: Karklins, Karlis (ed.). *Studies in Material Culture Research*. Uniontown: The Society for Historical Archaeology.
Durning, Louise. (2009). The Oxford college as household, 1590–1640. In: Cavallo, Sandra and Evangelisti, Silvia (eds). *Domestic Institutional Interiors in Early Modern Europe*. Farnham: Ashgate.

Edington, Barry. (2007). A space for moral management: The York Retreat's influence on asylum design. In: Topp, Leslie Elizabeth, Moran, James E., and Andrews, Jonathan (eds). *Madness, Architecture and the Built Environment: Psychiatric Spaces in Historical Context*. London: Routledge.

Ellis, Robert. (2001). A field of practice or a mere house of detention? The asylum and its integration, with special reference to the county asylums of Yorkshire, c.1844–1888. Doctor of Philosophy, University of Huddersfield.

__ (2008). The asylum, the Poor Law and the growth of county asylums in nineteenth-century Yorkshire. *Northern History* 45(2): 279–293.

Ellis, W.C. (1838). *A Treatise on the Nature, Symptoms, Causes, and Treatment of Insanity*. London: Samuel Holdsworth.

Elsner, John. (2004). A collector's model of desire: The House and museum of Sir John Soane. In: Cardinal, Roger (ed.). *Cultures of Collecting*. London: Reaktion Books.

Epperson, Terrence W. (2000). Panoptic plantations: the garden sights of Thomas Jefferson and George Mason. In: Delle, James A., Mrozowski, Stephen A., and Paynter, Robert (eds). *Lines that Divide: Historical Archaeologies of Race, Class and Gender*. Knoxville: University of Tennessee Press.

Evans, Timothy H. (2004). Tradition and illusion: Antiquarianism, tourism and horror in H.P. Lovecraft. *Extrapolation* 45(2): 176–195.

Feld, Steve and Brenneis, Donald. (2004). Doing anthropology in sound. *American Ethnologist* 31(4): 461–474.

Fennelly, Katherine. (2014). Out of sound, out of mind: noise control in early nineteenth-century lunatic asylums in England and Ireland. *World Archaeology* 46(3): 416–430.

Field, Siân. (1994). 'Warehousing the unwanted': Moral architecture as applied to London County Council Lunatic Asylum, with specific reference to Claybury Asylum, Essex. BSc Thesis, University College London.

Finnane, Mark. (1981). *Insanity and the Insane in Post-famine Ireland*. London: Croom Helm.

First Report: Minutes of Evidence Taken Before the Select Committee Appointed to Consider of Provision being made for the Better Regulation of Madhouses, in England; 1815 (227).

Fogerty, William. (1867). On the planning of lunatic asylums. *The Irish Builder* 9(172): 39–40.

Foljambe, J. (1814). To Architects. West Riding of Yorkshire. *Leeds Mercury*, 17 December 1814.

Foucault, Michel. (1991). *Discipline and Punish: the Birth of the Prison*. London: Penguin.

__ (2006). *Madness and Civilization; a History of Insanity in the Age of Reason*. London: Routledge.

__ and Miskowiec, Jay. (1986). Of other spaces. *Diacritics* 16(1): 22–27.

Franklin, Bridget. (2002a). Hospital – heritage – home: Reconstructing the nineteenth century lunatic asylum. *Housing, Theory and Society* 19(3–4): 170–184

__ (2002b). Monument to madness: the rehabilitation of the Victorian lunatic asylum. *Journal of Architectural Conservation* 8(3): 24–39.

Franklin, Jill. (1981). *The Gentleman's Country House and its Plan. 1835–1914*. London: Routledge and Kegan Paul.

Furján, Helene. (1997). The specular spectacle of the house of the collector. *Assemblage* (34): 57–91.
Geary, Laurence M. (2004). *Medicine and Charity in Ireland 1718–1851*. Dublin: University College Dublin Press.
Geber, Jonny. (2015). *Victims of Ireland's Great Famine: The Bioarchaeology of Mass Burial at Kilkenny Union Workhouse*. Gainesville: University Press of Florida.
Gieryn, Thomas F. (2001). What buildings do. *Theory and Society* 31(1): 35–74.
Giles, Katherine and Giles, Melanie. (2010). Signs of the times: Nineteenth–twentieth century graffiti in the farms of the Yorkshire Wolds. *Studies in Contemporary and Historical Archaeology (BAR S2074)* 6: 47–59.
Girouard, Mark. (1978). *Life in the English Country House*. New Haven: Yale University Press.
Goffman, Erving. (1976). *Asylums: Essays on the Social Situation of Mental Patients and Other Inmates*. Middlesex: Penguin.
Goldberg, Ann. (1998). The Eberback Asylum and the practice(s) of nymphomania in Germany, 1815–1849. *Journal of Women's History* 9(4): 35–52.
Gore, Tony and Jones, Catherine. (2006). Yorkshire and the Humber. In: Hardill, Irene, et al. (eds). *The Rise of the English Regions?* Oxford: Routledge.
Government of Ireland. (2006). *A Vision for Change: Report of the Expert Group on Mental Health Policy*. Dublin: The Stationery Office.
Gray, Peter. (2004). Political economy and the memory of the great famine. In: Gray, Peter (ed.). *Victoria's Ireland? Irishness and Britishness, 1837–1901*. Dublin: Four Courts Press.
Greally, Hanna. (2009). *Bird's Nest Soup*. Cork: Attic Press.
Greenia, George D. (2005). The bigger the book: On oversize medieval manuscripts. *Revue belge de philologie et d'histoire* 83(3): 723–745.
Grimes, Kyle. (2008). *Fragments – Hone and the London Asylum (1813–1814)* [Online]. Available: http://honearchive.org/biographical/fragments/london-asylum.html [Accessed 23 September 2011].
Grimsley-Smith, Melinda. (2011). Politics, professionalization, and poverty: lunatic asylums for the poor in Ireland, 1817–1920. Doctor of Philosophy, Notre Dame.
__ (2012). Revisiting a 'demographic freak': Irish asylums and hidden hunger. *Social History of Medicine* 25(2): 307–323.
Guyatt, Mary. (2004). A semblance of home: Mental asylum interiors, 1880–1914. In: McKellar, Susie and Sparke, Penny (eds). *Interior Design and Identity*. Manchester: Manchester University Press.
Hallaran, William Saunders. (1818). *Practical Observations on the Causes and Cure of Insanity*. Cork: Edwards and Savage.
Hamilton, Sue, Whitehouse, Ruth, Brown, Keri, Combes, Pamela, Herring, Edward, and Thomas, Mike Seager. (2006). Phenomenology in practice: Towards a methodology for a 'subjective' approach. *European Journal of Archaeology* 9(1): 31–71.
Hamlett, Jane. (2015). *At Home in the Institution: Material life in Asylums, Lodging Houses and Schools in Victorian and Edwardian England*. London: Palgrave Macmillan.

__ and Hoskins, Lesley (2012). 'A bright and cheerful aspect': Wall decoration and the treatment of mental illness in the nineteenth and early twentieth centuries. *Wallpaper History Review* 11: 42–25.

Harvey, Robert. (2007). *The War of Wars: The Epic Struggle between Britain and France: 1789–1815*. London: Constable.

Hatton, Edward. (1708). *A New View of London; or, an Ample Account of that City, in Two Volumes, or Eight Sections: Volume Two*. London: John Nicholson, and Robert Knaplock.

Hewitt, Martin. (2000). Confronting the modern city: The Manchester Free Public Library. *Urban History* 27: 62–88.

Higginbotham, Peter. (2008). *The Workhouse Cookbook*. Stroud: The History Press.

Hill, Robert Gardiner. (1857). *A Concise History of the Entire Abolition of Mechanical Restraint in the Treatment of the Insane, and of the Introduction, Success and Final Triumph of the Non-restraint System*. London: Longman.

Hillier, Bill and Hanson, Julienne. (1984). *The Social Logic of Space*. Cambridge: Cambridge University Press.

Hilmes, Michele. (2005). Is there a field called sound culture studies? And does it matter? *American Quarterly* 57(1): 249–259.

Hine, George T. (1901). Asylums and asylum planning. *Journal of the RIBA* 8: 161–184.

Hume, Ivor Noël. (1964). Handmaiden to history. *North Carolina Historical Review* 41(2): 215–225.

Ingold, Tim. (1993). The temporality of the landscape. *World Archaeology* 25(2): 152–174.

Irish Architectural Archive: Holybrooke Drawings Collection.

Irish Architectural Archive: Murray Collection of Architectural Drawings.

Irish Architectural Archive: Wilkinson Collection of Workhouse Drawings.

Jackson, Alvin. (1999). *Ireland 1798–1998: Politics and War*. Oxford: Blackwell.

Jacob, John. (1833). *Observations and Suggestions on the Management of Maryborough District Lunatic Asylum*. Dublin: P. Dixon Hardy.

Jacobi, Maximilian. (1841). *On the Construction and Management of Hospitals for the Insane: with a Particular Notice of the Institution at Siegburg*. London: John Churchill.

Jones, Declan. (1990). History and theory dissertation: St. Ita's Hospital, Portrane. Thesis, University College Dublin.

Joseph, Alun, Kearns, Robin, and Moon, Graham. (2013) Re-imagining psychiatric asylum spaces through residential redevelopment: Strategic forgetting and selective remembrance. *Housing Studies* 28(1): 135–153.

Joyce, Patrick. (2003). *The Rule of Freedom: Liberalism and the Modern City*. London: Verso.

Kearns, Gerry. (2006). Dublin, modernity and the postcolonial spatial fix. *Irish Geography* 39(2): 177–183.

Kelly, B. (2004). Mental illness in 19th century Ireland: A qualitative study of Workhouse Records. *Irish Journal of Medical Science* 173(1): 53–55.

__ (2008a). Dr William Saunders Hallaran and psychiatric practice in nineteenth-century Ireland. *Irish Journal of Medical Science* 177(1): 79–84.

___ (2008b). Mental health law in Ireland, 1821 to 1902: Building the asylums. *Medico-Legal Journal* 76(1): 19–25.

___ (2014). *Custody, Care and Criminality: Forensic Psychiatry and Law in 19th Century Ireland.* Dublin: The History Press Ireland.

Kennihan, Ryan. (2003). On an asylum: A brief history lesson followed by some reflections on a peculiar section and its inherent myth. *Building Material* 10: 50–59.

Kincaid, Andrew. (2006). *Postcolonial Dublin: Imperial Legacies and the Built Environment.* London: University of Minnesota Press.

King, Stacie M. and Santiago, Gonzalo Sanchez. (2011). Soundscapes of the everyday in ancient Oaxaca, Mexico. *Archaeologies: Journal of the World Archaeological Congress* 7: 387–422.

Kirby, Mike. (2008). *SE3320: Caleb Crowther Almshouses – George Street* [Online]. Available: www.geograph.org.uk/photo/937648 [Accessed 26 January 2012].

Laffey, Paul. (2003). Psychiatric therapy in Georgian Britain. *Psychological Medicine* 33: 1285–1297.

Lennon, John and Foley, Malcolm. (2000). *Dark Tourism: The Attraction of Death and Disaster.* Padstow: Continuum.

Leone, Mark P. (1995). A historical archaeology of capitalism. *American Anthropologist* 97(2): 251–268.

Levine-Clark, Marjorie. (2004). 'Embarrassed circumstances': Gender, poverty, and insanity in the West Riding of England in the mid Victorian years. In: Andrews, Jonathan and Digby, Ann (eds). *Sex and Seclusion. Class and Custody. Perspectives on Gender and Class in the History of British and Irish Psychiatry.* Amsterdam: Rodopi.

Levitt, Sarah and Tozer, Jane. (1983 [2010]). *Fabric of Society: a Century of People and their Clothes 1770–1870. Essays Inspired by the Collections at Platt Hall, The Gallery of Costume, Manchester.* Manchester: Manchester Art Gallery, Manchester Art Gallery Trust, and Manchester City Council.

Lewis, Samuel. (1837). *A Topographical Dictionary of Ireland: Comprising the Several Counties, Cities, Boroughs, Corporate, Market and Post Towns. Parishes and Villages, with Historical and Statistical Description.* London: S. Lewis & Co.

Longford, Elizabeth. (1985). 194: Duchess of Richmond's ball. In: Hastings, Max (ed.). *The Oxford Book of Military Anecdotes.* Oxford: Oxford University Press.

Longhurst, Peta. (2015). Institutional non-correspondence: Materiality and ideology in the mental institutions of New South Wales. *Post-Medieval Archaeology* 49(2): 220–237.

Louden, John Claudius. (1846). *Encyclopaedia of Cottage, Farm, and Villa Architecture and Furniture.* London: Longman, Brown, Green and Longmans.

Lovecraft, H.P. (2011). *The Call of Cthulu and Other Weird Stories.* London: Penguin.

___ (2018). *The Thing on the Doorstep* [ebook]. Oregan Publishing.

Lucas, Gavin. (1999). The archaeology of the workhouse: changing uses of the workhouse buildings at St. Mary's, Southampton. In: Tarlow, Sarah and West, Susie (eds). *The Familiar Past: Archaeologies of Later Historical Britain.* London: Routledge.

Luddy, Maria. (2007). *Prostitution and Irish Society, 1800–1940*. Cambridge: Cambridge University Press.
M'Cready, C.T. (1987). *Dublin Street Names: Dated and Explained (reprint)*. Dublin: Carraig Books Ltd.
Macalpine, Ida and Hunter, Richard. (1991). *George III and the Mad-Business*. London: Pimlico.
MacKinnon, Dolly. (2003). Hearing madness: The soundscapes of the asylum. In: Coleborne, Catharine and Mackinnon, Dolly (eds). *'Madness' in Australia: Histories, Heritage and the Asylum*. Queensland: University of Queensland Press.
__ (2011). Snatches of music, flickering images and the smell of leather: The material culture of recreational pastimes in psychiatric collections in Scotland and Australia. In: Colebourne, Catharine and Mackinnon, Dolly (eds). *Exhibiting Madness in Museums: Remembering Psychiatry through Collections and Display*. London: Routledge.
Markus, Thomas A. (1982). Building for the sad, the bad and the mad in urban Scotland, 1780–1830. In: Markus, Thomas A. (ed.). *Order in Space and Society: Architectural Form and its context in the Scottish Enlightenment*. Edinburgh: Mainstream Publishing Company Ltd.
__ (1983). Buildings and the ordering of minds and bodies. In: Jones, Peter (ed.). *Philosophy and Science in the Scottish Enlightenment*. Edinburgh: John Donald Publishers Ltd.
__ (1989). Class and classification in the buildings of the late Scottish Enlightenment. In: Devine, T.M. (ed.). *Improvement and Enlightenment: Proceedings of the Scottish Historical Studies Seminar. University of Strathclyde 1987–88*. Edinburgh: John Donald Publishers Ltd.
__ (1993). *Buildings and Power: Freedom and Control in the Origin of Modern Building Types*. London; New York: Routledge.
Marland, Hilary. (1987). *Medicine and Society in Wakefield and Huddersfield: 1780–1870*. Cambridge: Cambridge University Press.
Matthews, Christopher and Palus, Matthew. (2007). A landscape of ruins: Building historical Annapolis. In: Hicks, Dan, McAtackney, Laura, and Fairclough, Graham (eds). *Envisioning Landscape: Situations and Standpoints in Archaeology and Heritage*. Walnut Creek: West Coast Press.
McAtackney, Laura. (2014). *An Archaeology of the Troubles: The Dark Heritage of Long Kesh/Maze Prison*. Oxford: Oxford University Press.
McHugh, Roger. (1949). *Carlow in '98: the Autobiography of William Farrell of Carlow*. Dublin: The Richview Press.
McKenzie, D.F. (2002). The book as an expressive form. In: Finkelstein, David and McCleery, Alistair (eds). *The Book History Reader*. Oxford: Routledge.
Meehan, Bernard. (2009). *The Book of Kells: An Illustrated Introduction to the Manuscript in Trinity College Dublin*. London: Thames and Hudson.
Middleton, Charles. (1810). *Decorations for Parks and Gardens: Designs for Gates, Garden Seats, Alcoves, Temples, Baths, Entrance Gates, Lodges, Facades, Prospect Towers, Cattle Sheds, Ruins, Bridges, Greenhouses, &c. &c. also a Hot House & Hot Wall: With Plans & Scales on 55 Plates*. London: J. Taylor.
Miller, John. (1878). *The Country Gentleman's Architect, in a Great Variety of New Designs*. London: J. Taylor.

Miller, Kerby A. (1988). *Emigrants and Exiles: Ireland and the Irish Exodus to North America*. Oxford: Oxford University Press.
Miron, Janet. (2011). *Prisons, Asylums and the Public: Institutional Visiting in the Nineteenth Century*. Toronto: University of Toronto Press.
Monk, Lee-Ann. (2003). Gender, space and work: The asylum as gendered workplace in Victoria. In: Coleborne, Catharine and Mackinnon, Dolly (eds). *'Madness' in Australia: Histories, Heritage and the Asylum*. Queensland: Queensland University Press.
Moore, J.E. (1967). *Design for Good Acoustics*. 2nd edn. London: Architectural Press.
Morrison, Kathryn. (1999). *The Workhouse: A Study of Poor-Law Buildings in England*. Swindon: Royal Commission on the Historical Monuments of England.
Mowl, Timothy. (1984). The evolution of the park gate lodge as a building type. *Architectural History* 27: 467–480.
Mytum, H. (2013). Materiality matters: The role of things in coping strategies at Cunningham's Camp, Douglas during World War I. In: Mytum, H. and Carr, G. (eds). *Prisoners of War: Archaeology, Memory, and Heritage of 19th- and 20th-Century Mass Internment*. New York: Springer.
__ and Carr, G. (eds). (2013). *Prisoners of War: Archaeology, Memory, and Heritage of 19th- and 20th-Century Mass Internment*. New York: Springer.
National Archives of Ireland, Dublin: Chief Secretary's Office Registered Papers (CSO/RP).
National Archives of Ireland: Cholera Papers for Queen's County 1832–33 (CP 2/440/9).
National Archives of Ireland: Plans of the Richmond Asylum, 1897–1901 (OPW 5HC/4/799).
National Archives of Ireland: Plans of Clonmel Asylum (OPW 5HC/4/884).
National Archives of Ireland: Commissioners for General Control and Correspondence for Superintending and Directing the Erection, Establishment and Regulation of Asylums for the Lunatic Poor in Ireland. Private Accession. (OPW 999/784).
National Archives of Ireland: Richmond District Lunatic Asylum Minute Books.
National Inventory of Architectural Heritage. (2019). Saint Senan's Psychiatric Hospital originally Wexford County Lunatic Asylum, Enniscorthy, County Wexford - 15604052. [Online]. Available: www.buildingsofireland.ie/niah/search.jsp?type=record&county=WX&regno=15604052 [Accessed 17 January 2019].
National Library of Ireland: Diary of Francis Johnston. Architect. 25 March–14 April 1796. Geacological Notes. MS/2722.
Newman, Charlotte. (2013). An archaeology of poverty: architectural innovation and pauper experience at Madeley Union Workhouse, Shropshire. *Post-Medieval Archaeology* 47(2): 359–377.
__ (2015). A mansion for the mad: an archaeology of Brooke House, Hackney. *Post-Medieval Archaeology* 49(1): 156–174.
__ (2016). Poverty and illness in the 'Old Countries': Archaeological approaches to historical medical institutions in the British Isles. *International Journal of Historical Archaeology* 21(1): 178–197.

Nolan, Peter W. (1993). A history on the training of asylum nurses. *Journal of Advanced Nursing* 18(8): 1193–1201.

Noll, Richard. (2007). *Encyclopaedia of Schizophrenia*. 3rd edn. New York: Facts on File, Inc.

Nord, Deborah Epstein. (1988). The city as theatre: From Georgian to Early Victorian London. *Victorian Studies* 31(2): 159–188.

O' Brien, Gerard. (1986). Workhouse management in pre-famine Ireland. *Proceedings of the Royal Irish Academy. Section C: Archaeology, Celtic Studies, History, Linguistics, Literature* 86C: 113–134.

O'Connor, J. (1992). *The Workhouses of Ireland: The Fate of Ireland's Poor*. Dublin: Mercer.

O'Donnell, P.D. (1972). Dublin Military Barracks. *Dublin Historical Record* 25(4): 141–154.

Ó Gráda, Cormac. (1993). *Before and After the Famine: Explorations in Economic History, 1800–1925*. 2nd edn. Manchester: Manchester University Press.

__ (1999). *Black '47 and Beyond: The Great Irish Famine in History, Economy, and Memory*. Woodstock: Princeton University Press.

O'Néill, Diarmuid. (2005). *Rebuilding the Celtic Languages: Reversing Language Shift in the Celtic Countries*. Ceredigion: Y Lolfa.

Ordnance Survey County Series 1st Edition. Published 1837–42. Ordnance Survey of Ireland, Dublin. Using: Ordnance Survey Ireland, http://maps.osi.ie [Accessed January 2017].

Orser, Charles E. (2007). *The Archaeology of Race and Racialization in Historic America*. Gainesville: University Press of Florida.

Parry-Jones, W.L. (1972). *The Trade in Lunacy: A Study of Private Madhouses in England in the Eighteenth and Nineteenth Centuries*. London: Routledge and Kegan Paul.

Pauls, Elizabeth P. (2006). The place of space: Architecture, landscape and social life. In: Hall, Martin and Silliman, Stephen W. (eds). *Historical Archaeology*. Oxford: Blackwell Publishing.

Payne, Christopher, and Sacks, Oliver. (2009). *Asylum: Inside the Closed World of State Mental Hospitals*. London: MIT Press.

Philo, Chris. (2004). *A Geographical History of Institutional Provision for the Insane from Medieval Times to the 1860's in England and Wales*. Lewiston: Edwin Mellen Press.

Piddock, Susan. (2007). *A Space of their Own: The Archaeology of Nineteenth-century Lunatic Asylums in Britain, South Australia and Tasmania*. New York: Springer.

__ (2009). John Conolly's 'ideal' asylum and provisions for the insane in nineteenth century South Australia and Tasmania. In: Beisaw, April M. and Gibb, James G. (eds). *The Archaeology of Institutional Life*. Tuscaloosa: University of Alabama Press.

Pinel, Phillippe. (1806). *A Treatise on Insanity*. London: Mssrs Cadell and Davis.

Porter, Roy. (1995). *Medicine in the Enlightenment*. Amsterdam: Rodopi Bv Editions.

__ (2001). *Enlightenment*. London: Penguin.

__ (2002). *Madness: a Brief History*. Oxford: Oxford University Press.

__ (2004). *Madmen: a Social History of Madhouses, Mad-doctors and Lunatics*. Stroud: Tempus Publishing Limited.
Powell, E. (1961). 'Water Tower Speech.' [Online]. Available: http://studymore.org.uk/xpowell.htm [Accessed 15 December 2017].
Prior, Lindsay. (1988). The architecture of the hospital: a study of spatial organisation and medical knowledge. *British Journal of Sociology* 39(1): 86–113.
Prior, Pauline (ed.) (2012). *Asylums, Mental Health Care, and the Irish, 1800–2010*. Newbridge: Irish Academic Press.
Pritchard, Allan. (1991). The urban gothic of *Bleak House*. *Nineteenth-Century Literature* 45(4): 432–452.
Psota, Sunshine. (2011). the archaeology of mental illness from the afflicted and caretaker perspective: A Northern California family's odyssey. *Historical Archaeology* 45(4): 20–38.
Rees, Rosemary. (2001). *Poverty and Public Health 1815–1948*. Oxford: Heinemann Educational Publishers.
Registry of Deeds for the Republic of Ireland: Deeds for land sold to Commissioners of Lunacy, Maryborough (865-184-58614).
Report from the Committee on Madhouses in England; 1815 (296).
Report from the Select Committee Appointed to Enquire into the State of Lunatics; 1808 (39).
Report on the District, Local, and Private Lunatic Asylums in Ireland, 1845: with appendices; 1846 (736).
Reuber, Markus. (1996). The architecture of psychological management: The Irish asylums (1801–1922). *Psychological Medicine* 26(6): 1179–1189.
Reynolds, Joseph. (1992). *Grangegorman: Psychiatric Care in Dublin since 1815*. Dublin: Institute of Public Administration.
Richardson, H. (1992). *Kent, Dartford, Bexley, Old Bexley Lane, Bexley Hospital. Virtual Catalogue Entry to support E.I. Migration*. [Online]. Available: http://archaeologydataservice.ac.uk/archsearch/record?titleId=1877651 [Accessed 23 December 2017].
Richardson, Harriet (ed.) (1998). *English Hospitals 1660–1948: A Survey of Their Architecture and Design*. Swindon: Royal Commission on the Historical Monuments of England.
Robins, Joseph. (1986). *Fools and Mad: a History of the Insane in Ireland*. Dublin: Institute of Public Administration.
Rose, Marice. (2011). *Kells to Clonmacnoise: Medieval Irish Art in Context Didactics*. Fairfield: Bellarmine Museum of Art.
Rutherford, Sarah. (2005). Landscapes for the mind: English asylum designers, 1845–1914. *Garden History* 33(1): 61–86.
__ (2008). *The Victorian Asylum*. Oxford: Shire Publications.
Sabine, Joseph. (1823). On the native country of the wild potato, with an account of its culture in the garden of the Horticultural Society; and Observations on the importance of obtaining improved varieties of the cultivated plant. *The Quarterly Journal of Science, Literature and the Arts* 15: 259.
Saeedi, Pouneh. (2009). Images of liminality in Book VI of *The Aeneid*. *Comparative Literature and Culture* 11(2): 8.
Sala, George Augustus. (1859). *Gaslight and Daylight with some London scenes they shine upon*. London: Chapman and Hall.

Scarre, Chris and Lawson, Graeme (eds). (2006). *Archaeoacoustics*. Cambridge: McDonald Institute for Archaeological Research.
Schofield, John and Graves-Brown, Paul. (2011). The filth and the fury: 6 Denmark Street (London) and the Sex Pistols. *Antiquity* 85(330): 1985–1401.
Schwartz, Hillel. (2004). On noise. In: Smith, Mark M. (ed.) *Hearing History: A Reader*. London: The University of Georgia Press.
Scull, Andrew. (1989). *Social Order / Mental Disorder: Anglo-American Psychiatry in Historical Perspective*. Berkeley: University of California Press.
__ (1993). *The Most Solitary of Afflictions: Madness and Society in Britain, 1700–1900*. New Haven: Yale University Press.
Select Committee on State of Gaols, and Best Method of Providing for Reformation of Offenders. Report, Minutes of Evidence, Appendix; 1819 (579).
Semple, Janet. (1993). *Bentham's Prison: A Study of the Panopticon Penitentiary*. Oxford: Oxford University Press.
Shackleford, Steve (ed.). (2009). *Blades Guide to Knives and Their Values: The Complete Handbook of Knife Collecting*. Iola: Krause Publications.
Shaw-Taylor, Leigh (2007). Diverse experiences: The geography of adult female employment in England and the 1851 Census. In: Goose, Nigel (ed.) *Women's Work in Industrial England: Regional and Local Perspectives*. Hatfield: Local Population Studies.
Sheahan, Patrick and Clery, Timothy. (1933). Portlaoighse Mental Hospital Laoighse: Extension to Dining Hall, Erection of Two Verandas. Limerick: Architects and Civil Engineers.
Showalter, Elaine. (1980). Victorian women and insanity. *Victorian Studies* 23(2): 157–181.
Skae, David. (1863). A rational and practical classification of insanity. *British Journal of Psychiatry* 47(9): 309–319.
Skrdla, Harry. (2006). *Ghostly Ruins: America's Forgotten Architecture*. New York: Princeton Architectural Press.
Smith, Adam. (1776). *An Inquiry into the Nature and Causes of the Wealth of Nations*. London: W. Strahan.
Smith, Leonard D. (1988). Behind closed doors: Lunatic asylum keepers, 1800–60. *Social History of Medicine* 1(3): 301–327.
__ (1995). The 'Great Experiment': The place of Lincoln in the history of psychiatry. *Lincolnshire History and Archaeology* 30: 55–62.
__ (1999). *'Cure, Comfort and Safe Custody.' Public Lunatic Asylums in Early Nineteenth Century England*. London: Leicester University Press.
__ (2007). The architecture of confinement: Urban public asylums in England, 1750–1820. In: Topp, Leslie Elizabeth, Moran, James E., and Andrews, Jonathan (eds). *Madness, Architecture and the Built Environment: Psychiatric Spaces in Historical Context*. London: Routledge.
Snaith, R.P. (1998). Images in psychiatry: The West Riding Pauper Lunatic Asylum. *American Journal of Psychiatry* 155(4): 456.
Stallard, Joshua Harrison. (1865). *Workhouse Hospitals*. London: L. Booth.
Stanley Royd Hospital: digital archive dedicated to the former Pauper Lunatic Asylum, Wakefield [Online]. Available: www.stanleyroydhospital.co.uk/ [Accessed 4 September 2012].
Stark, William. (1810). *Remarks on the construction of public hospitals for the*

cure of mental derangement: read to a committee of inhabitants of the city of Glasgow, appointed to receive plans, with a view to that object. Glasgow: James Hedderwick and Co.

Stephens, W.B. (1987). *Education, Literacy and Society, 1830–70.* Manchester: Manchester University Press.

Stevenson, Christine. (2000). *Medicine and Magnificence: British Hospital and Asylum Architecture, 1660–1815.* London: Yale University Press.

Stone, Philip R. (2006). A dark tourism spectrum: Towards a typology of death and macabre related tourist sites, attractions and exhibitions. *Tourism: An Interdisciplinary International Journal* 54(2): 145–60.

St. Patrick's Hospital Archives, Dublin: Plan No. 2 by Francis Johnston, 1817 (F/8).

St. Patrick's Hospital Archives, Dublin: Plan for a Laundry by William Murray (F/9).

Tarlow, Sarah. (2007). *The Archaeology of Improvement, 1750–1850.* Cambridge: Cambridge University Press.

Taylor, Jeremy. (1991). *Hospital and Asylum Architecture in England, 1840–1914: Building for Health Care.* London: Mansell.

__ (1995). The architectural image of the asylum. *The Victorian Society Annual 1995.* London: the Victorian Society.

Till, Rupert. (2011). *Sounds of Stonehenge* [Online]. Wordpress. Available: http://soundsofstonehenge.wordpress.com/methodology/ [Accessed 20 September 2011].

The Census of Ireland for the year 1851. Part IV. Report on Ages and Education. 1856 (2053).

The Forty-Seventh Report (with appendices) of the Inspectors of Lunatics (Ireland); 1898 (8969).

The National Archives of the United Kingdom: Audits of Maryborough District Lunatic Asylum 1842–66 (AO 19/48/14).

The National Archives of the United Kingdom: Audits of Richmond District Lunatic Asylum 1842–67 (AO 19/48/17).

The National Archives of the United Kingdom: Commissioners for Auditing the Public Accounts, 1833–34 (AO 2/68–70).

Thomas, J. (2009). *Gateway to Rise Hall* [Online]. Available: www.geograph.org.uk/photo/1467836 [Accessed 15 February 2012].

Thompson, John D. and Goldin, Grace. (1975). *The Hospital: A Social and Architectural History.* New Haven: Yale University Press.

Topp, Leslie Elizabeth, Moran, James E., and Andrews, Jonathan (eds). (2007). *Madness, Architecture and the Built Environment: Psychiatric Spaces in Historical Context,* New York; London: Routledge.

Tucker, Kathryn Maeder. (2007). Theatre as asylum, asylum as theatre: Cross-channel institutional intersections from 1780 to 1830. Doctor of Philosophy, University of California.

Tuke, Samuel. (1813). *Description of the Retreat, an institution near York for Insane Persons of the Society of Friends.* York: W. Alexander.

__ (1819). Practical hints on the construction and economy of pauper lunatic asylums. In: Watson, Charles and Pritchett, James Pigott (eds). *Plans, Elevations and Sections and Description of the Pauper Lunatic Asylum lately erected at Wakefield.* 2nd edn. York: W. Alexander.

Turner, Victor W. (1969). *The Ritual Process: Structure and Anti-Structure*. London: Routledge and Kegan Paul.
Van Gennep, Arnold. (1960). *The Rites of Passage*. Chicago: University of Chicago Press.
Veis, Nurin. (2011). The ethics of exhibiting psychiatric materials. In: Coleborne, Catharine and Mackinnon, Dolly (eds). *Exhibiting Madness in Museums: Remembering Psychiatry through Collections and Display*. London: Routledge.
Vickery, Amanda. (2009). *Behind Closed Doors: At Home in Georgian England*. London: Yale University Press.
Vince, Alan. (2003). Lincoln in the early modern era (c.1350-c.1750). In: Stocker, David (ed.). *The City by the Pool: Assessing the Archaeology of the City of Lincoln*. Oxford: Oxbow.
Vincent, David. (1993). *Literacy and Popular Culture: England 1750–1914*. Cambridge: Cambridge University Press.
Wakefield, Edward. (1812). *An Account of Ireland, Statistical and Political*. London: Longman, Hurst, Rees, Orme, and Brown.
Walsh, Claire. (2001). The City Workhouse, St. James's Hospital, St. James Street, Dublin. Excavations 0137338; OOE647.
Walsh, Oonagh. (1997). 'A lightness of mind': Gender and insanity in nineteenth century Ireland. In: Kelleher, Margaret and Murphy, James H. (eds). *Gender Perspectives in Nineteenth Century Ireland: Public and Private Spheres*. Dublin: Irish Academic Press.
Ward, Eilis. (2006). Security and asylum: The case of Hanna Greally. *Studies: An Irish Quarterly Review* 95(377): 65–76.
Watson, Aaron and Keating, David. (1999). Architecture and sound: An acoustic analysis of megalithic monuments in Prehistoric Britain. *Antiquity* 73: 325–336.
Watson, Charles and Pritchett, James Pigott (eds). (1819). *Plans, Elevations, Sections, and Description of the Pauper Lunatic Asylum at Wakefield, To Which is Added a New and Enlarged Edition of S. Tuke's Practical Hints on the Construction and Economy of Pauper Lunatic Asylums*, York.
Weldrake, Dave. (2012). *Identifying your Finds: A Beginner's Guide to What to Look For. First Steps in Identifying and Dating Clay Tobacco Pipes*. [Online]. Wakefield: West Yorkshire Archaeology Advisory Service. Available: www.archaeology.wyjs.org.uk/wyjs-archaeology-identifying-r.asp [Accessed 4 May 2012].
West Yorkshire Archives Service, Wakefield: Departments Catalogue, Clerk of the Peace Records (QD1).
West Yorkshire Archives Service, Wakefield: West Riding Pauper Lunatic Asylum (C85).
White, S.D. (2015). Clay Tobacco Pipes. In: Andrews, Phil (ed.). *Riverside Exchange, Sheffield: Investigations on the Site of the Town Mill, Cutlers' Wheel, Marshall's Steelworks and the Naylor Vickers Works*. Salisbury: Oxbow.
White, R.J. (1957). *Waterloo to Peterloo*. Harmondsworth: Penguin.
Wilkie, Laurie. (2006). Documentary archaeology. In: Hicks, Dan and Beaudry, Mary (eds). *The Cambridge Companion to Historical Archaeology*. Cambridge: Cambridge University Press.
Williams, David. (1999). *The Enlightenment*. Cambridge: Cambridge University Press.

Williamson, Arthur P. (1976). Armagh District Lunatic Asylum: The first phase. *Seanchas Ardmhacha: Journal of the Armagh Diocesan Historical Society* 8(1): 111–120.

__ (1992). Psychiatry, moral management and the origins of social policy for mentally ill people in Ireland. *Irish Journal of Medical Science* 161(9): 556–558.

Williamson, T. (2007). Introduction: Archaeological perspectives on estate landscapes. In: Finch, Johnathan and Giles, Katherine (eds). *Estate Landscapes: Design, Improvement and Power in the Post-Medieval Landscape*. Woodbridge: The Boydell Press.

Woodham-Smith, Cecil. (1962). *The Great Hunger: Ireland 1845–1849*. London: H. Hamilton.

Yanni, Carla. (2007). *The Architecture of Madness: Insane Asylums in the United States*. Minneapolis: University of Minnesota Press.

Index

Abbott, William 41, 83, 105
Act of Union (1801) 70
administration
  and colonialism 70, 72
  material culture 27–31, 70–3, 94, 106, 113–14, 148
  paperwork 28–9, 83–5, 94–5, 104
  reform in the nineteenth century 72, 113
  stamps 89–90, 95, 109–10, 114
  wax seals 95, 114
administration block 73–97
  architecture 71, 73–5, 78–81, 83, 92–3
  living quarters 81, 93–4, 128
  and power 128, 131
admission 25, 92, 96–7, 100, 113, 139
  paperwork 83–5, 102
  process 71, 80–8, 97, 100–2, 147
  rates 56–7, 61
agency 16, 24, 28, 94, 143
Andover Workhouse 73
anti-psychiatry 15, 17
architecture of asylums
  arrangement 36–7, 45, 63, 69–70, 78–80, 82–3, 117–18, 136, 143
  influences 8, 11, 60, 74–5, 79, 97–101, 113, 116, 129, 131–2, 146–7
Arkham Asylum 22, 148
Armagh Lunatic Asylum 40, 43, 64, 84, 127–8, 143
attendants 47–8
  handbook 49
  see also keepers
Australia 3, 14, 25, 91, 111
  New South Wales 15
  Tasmania 18

Ballinasloe Lunatic Asylum 64
baths
  in the asylum 34, 56, 82–3, 85–7, 124, 127, 137, 139
  and the public 86
Battie, William 35
Belfast Lunatic Asylum 64, 127
Bentham, Jeremy 20, 118–20, 128, 131–2
Bethlem Hospital 6, 10, 35, 40–2, 47, 123
  Crossrail excavations 5
  Moorfields 5, 10
  Priory of St Mary Bethlehem 5
  St George's Fields 5, 42
Bevans, James 45, 60, 79, 80, 108, 122–7, 129
Bevans, John 36–7
Bexley Hospital 27
Bîcètre 35
Board of General Control 11–12, 39–40, 58, 78, 84, 94, 107, 123, 125–7
Bracebridge Heath *see* Lincolnshire County Asylum
British Medical Journal 43, 135
Brooke House, Chiswick 15
  see also Newman, Charlotte
Browne, W.A.F. 9, 48

Carlow Lunatic Asylum 69, 75, 76, 83, 93, 105, 128, 132, 136
Casella, Eleanor Conlin 28
Census (1851) 111
Charlesworth, Edward Parker 9, 34, 36, 42–3, 146, 150
Chelsea Hospital 8
cholera 66, 85
  outbreaks 67, 82

circulating swing 10, 36, 117
classification 5, 16, 24–5, 33–4, 38, 46, 56–8, 60–1, 75, 78, 80, 83, 100, 119–20, 126, 134–6, 138
Claybury Lunatic Asylum 78
clerks
  duties 94–5
  handwriting 94
  as individuals 71
  in the nineteenth century 94, 96
  spaces for 73, 94–6
Clonmel Lunatic Asylum 63, 102, 141
colleges, architecture of 100
Colney Hatch Asylum 150
commercial archaeology xiii, 23, 27, 153–4
  Grey literature 19
Commissioners of Lunacy
  creation of 10, 12
  reports of 71
Committee on Madhouses (1815)
  Haslam, John 40–2
  Monro, Thomas 40–2
  Norris, James William 41–2
Conolly, John 12, 34, 44, 48
  on asylum architecture 38, 115, 125, 145
  and Hanwell 38, 115
  on management 40, 44–5, 75, 146
  see also Hanwell; Middlesex County Asylum
Cooley, Thomas 11, 79
Cork City Asylum 9
Cork Lunatic Asylum 135
Cornwall County Asylum 75
Corsellis, Charles 39, 44–6, 48, 56–7, 82
County Asylums Act (1808) 10, 12, 106, 108, 151
County Asylums Act (1828) 10
Cox, Joseph Mason 36
  see also circulating swing; Fishponds
Crichton-Browne, James 46
Crooked Acres Hospital 27
Crowther, Caleb 39, 44–5 49, 88, 141
cupola 74, 77, 104, 127, 131
  clock 131

Danvers State Hospital 22, 148
  see also Arkham Asylum; Lovecraft, H.P.
dark heritage 13, 22, 149, 154
dark tourism 21–2, 154

demography
  Ireland 111
  surge in population 6, 55
  United Kingdom 55–6
Devon County Asylum 71
Dickens, Charles 51
documentary archives
  methods 14–15, 26–8
  problems with 3, 29, 46, 81, 83, 136
  use of 3, 18, 29, 139, 146
  see also administration
domestic institutions 8, 93–4, 97, 126, 128, 133
  comfort 9, 45
  interiors 20–1, 45, 119, 136, 146
Dublin 7–8, 29, 43, 52, 60, 80, 92–3, 100, 107–9, 112, 127, 139
Dublin House of Industry 11, 33, 50–2, 57–9, 84, 88, 99
Dublin Lying-in Hospital 8
Duke of Richmond *see* Lennox, Charles, 4th Duke of Richmond
dysentery 85

Earl of Kildare 8
Edinburgh 7, 24, 52
Ellis, William
  Hanwell 44, 64
  Wakefield 36, 44
English Heritage 15, 27
Enlightenment 6–7, 9
Enniscorthy Asylum *see* Wexford County Lunatic Asylum
Esquirol, Jean-Étienne 9
Exe Vale Asylum *see* Devon County Asylum

famine in Ireland 19, 64–7, 72, 82, 91
Farrell, William 69, 105
female refuge 87
Fishponds 36
Fitzgerald, James *see* Earl of Kildare
food
  ceramics 109–10
  diet 19, 64–6
  starvation 64, 67
  utensils 89–90
Foucault, Michel 16–17, 20, 86, 117
  Discipline and Punish 116
  Great Confinement 6–7, 52
  on the imperative of labour 17
  Madness and Civilisation 6–7, 16, 86

Index

Gaelige, language 110–11
gamma maps
  definition 24
  use of 117, 139–40
Gandon, James 80, 123
Gandy, John 123
gate lodge 23, 25, 71, 80, 97–105, 113–14, 140–1, 146
  keepers 69, 96–9, 102, 104–5, 113–14, 147
  see also porter's lodge
gender 5, 16, 33, 47, 56–8, 61, 119, 144
George the Third, madness of 4, 35, 38
Georgian Order 6–8, 32–3, 36, 57, 62, 73–5, 78, 80, 114, 116,–17, 120, 131, 133, 138, 144
  see also Wide Streets Commission improvements
Glasgow Lunatic Asylum 135
  architecture 75, 119–20, 127
Goffman, Erving 15–17, 52, 71, 86, 88, 97, 101, 137
  see also anti-psychiatry; total institution
governor 57–8
  of the asylum 37, 94, 124, 128, 130, 140
Grangegorman Mental Hospital 151
  see also Richmond District Asylum

Hallaran, William Saunders 9–10, 34, 36, 117
  see also circulating swing; Cork City Asylum
Hanwell 12, 38, 44, 64, 88, 115
  see also Conolly, John, and Hanwell
Hardwick Fever Hospital 142
Hatton, Edward 8
Hill, Robert Gardiner 36, 43
Hine, G.T. 56, 78
Hume, Ivor Noël 27
hygiene
  hair-cutting 87–8
  see also baths

improvement, idea of 6–7, 52, 74, 80, 112
Inspector General of Prisons 10
institutional archaeology 14, 19
Ireland
  colonialism 91, 106, 110, 112, 114

Irish Builder, The 40
Irish Civil War 29, 112
Irish Commissioners of Lunacy 40
Irish Lunatic Asylums for the Poor Act (1817) 11–12, 106

Jackson, Alexander 43, 58
Jacob, John 41, 43, 45, 84, 88, 96, 102, 104, 133–4, 136
Jacobi, Maximilian 56
Johnston, Francis 78, 109, 125–8
  asylums 11, 40, 54, 58, 74–5, 78–9, 82, 85, 87, 92, 96, 127–9, 134–5, 137
  other works 52, 80, 99

keepers
  duties 23, 46–9, 53, 128, 130, 139, 144
  masculinity 47, 49
  neglect xi, 42, 47, 117, 121
  spaces 122, 124–5, 130
  uniform 132–3
  see also attendants
keys 23, 47, 104, 132–3
Kilkenny Union Workhouse 19, 66

laundry workers 46, 53, 69, 93
Lawn Asylum, The *see* Lincoln City Asylum
Lennox, Charles, 4th Duke of Richmond 75, 108–9, 112, 114
Limerick Lunatic Asylum 64, 127
liminality 25, 71, 73, 78, 86, 95, 97, 101, 105, 139
Lincoln City Asylum xiii, 18, 42–3, 62–3, 74, 108, 135
  non-restraint xiii, 9, 36, 42–3, 121
Lincoln Lunatic Asylum *see* Lincoln City Asylum
Lincolnshire County Asylum xiii, 63
literacy 51, 72, 83, 96, 105
Londonderry Lunatic Asylum 64
Lovecraft, H.P. 22, 148
Lunacy Acts (1845) 10, 12, 38, 68, 70, 72, 106–7, 115, 145

Macmillan, Harold 150
Madeley Union Workhouse 18
Madhouses Act (1828) 10
Magdalene asylums 16
  see also female refuge

Index

manager 12, 14, 37–41, 43–4, 46, 48–53, 61, 64, 67–8, 69–70, 72–3, 81–2, 84, 89, 91, 93–4, 96, 102, 104–5, 111, 113, 115–17, 121–2, 125, 127–8, 131, 133, 135, 139–41, 143, 147
  see also governor
Maryborough County Infirmary 66, 74, 92–3, 101, 108
Maryborough Gaol 66, 101, 108
Maryborough Lunatic Asylum xi, xiii, 32, 37, 41, 43, 65–7, 74–5, 77, 82–4, 88, 90, 91–3, 95, 101–5, 108–13, 132–4, 136–7, 139–141, 143–4
Mental Health Act (1959) 149
Mental Health Act (2001) 21, 151
Mental Treatment Act (1945) 151
Middlesex County Asylum 12, 38, 64, 88
  see also Hanwell
Monro, family of physicians 40
moral management 6, 8–10, 12, 24–5, 33–4, 36–41, 43–8, 50, 54–6, 60–2, 67–8, 74, 108, 115–6, 118, 120–1, 127–8, 131–2, 134, 144, 146–8
  see also traitment moral
Morning Star Avenue 99–100, 108, 140
Mullingar Lunatic Asylum see St Loman's Hospital
Murray, William 77, 103, 108, 131, 136–7
  and Johnston 63–4, 75, 92, 99, 127–8, 135

Napoleonic Wars 7–8, 49, 108
  veterans of 8, 49–50, 84
New Poor Law 74, 107
Newman, Charlotte 15, 18, 20–1
noise 25–6, 87, 120, 133–4, 136–8, 144
  see also sound
non-restraint xiii, 9, 12, 33, 34, 36, 38–9, 41–3, 45, 50, 58, 121
Nottinghamshire County Asylum 75
nurses 46–9, 51–2, 95, 104, 121, 130–1, 133, 136, 153
  see also attendants

Our Lady's Hospital 153
  see also Cork Lunatic Asylum
overcrowding xiii, 2, 5–6, 8, 11, 21, 32, 39, 45, 48, 54–68, 71, 117, 140–1, 155

panopticon 20, 116, 118–138, 144, 146–7
  definition 118–19
  see also Bentham, Jeremy
Peel, Robert 39, 78, 107–8, 112, 123
physician, role of 37, 39–41, 43–6, 48, 85–6, 88
Piddock, Susan xii, 14, 34
  see also institutional archaeology
Pinel, Phillippe 9, 17, 34–6
  see also Bîcètre
Planning for the Future 151
political economy 6, 72
Poor Law Commission 65, 73, 106
popular representations of asylums
  comics 148
  film 13, 21, 148, 156
  video games 21, 148–9
Porter, Roy 17
porter's lodge 98, 100
Portlaoighse Mental Hospital see Maryborough Lunatic Asylum
Powell, Enoch 24, 149–50
prisons xii, 4, 9, 13, 16, 18, 21, 32, 52, 55, 74, 117–19, 131, 133, 137–8, 144, 146–7, 155
  lunatics in 10–11
Pritchett, James Pigott see Watson and Pritchett
private asylums 4, 9, 10, 15, 20, 33–4, 36, 41, 44, 55–6, 59, 61, 63, 79, 85, 120, 126

Quakers 37

Rebellion (1798) 69, 112
redevelopment xiii, 13, 18, 21, 23, 27, 30–1, 53, 71, 113, 151–6
Renny, George 107
resistance 16–17, 53–4, 112
  archaeologies of 17–18, 53, 112
Richmond Bridewell 100
Richmond House of Correction 52
Richmond Lunatic Asylum 10–12, 43, 50–4, 57–60, 63–5, 75, 83–5, 87–8, 90, 95, 99–100, 102, 104, 107–9, 111–12, 126, 129, 131, 134–5, 137, 139–42, 144, 151
  see also Grangegorman Mental Hospital

Richmond Penitentiary 8, 50, 142
Rites of Passage, The 24, 71, 101
Roscommon Gaol 59, 78, 80, 107, 126–7
rules 16, 46, 49–53, 111

Semple, George 10, 79
sensory environment 26, 86, 137–8, 144, 147
　see also sound
Smith, Adam 6
smoking 49
　pipes 18, 90–1
Soane, John 123
Society of Friends *see* Quakers
sonic environment 26, 61, 133–4, 144
　see also sound
sound 25–6, 47, 132–8, 144
　see also noise
St Brendan's *see* Grangegorman Mental Hospital
St Ita's Hospital 145
St Loman's Hospital 88
St Luke's Hospital 35, 123
St Patrick's Hospital 10–11, 59, 79
St Senan's *see* Wexford County Lunatic Asylum
St John's *see* Lincolnshire County Asylum
Stanley Royd Hospital 152
　see also West Riding Asylum
Stark, William 80, 119–20, 127, 135
Stephen Beaumont Museum of Mental Health 27, 86, 89, 91, 135
stigma 13, 31, 151, 155–6
surveillance 25, 100–1, 116, 121, 126, 129–30, 138, 147
　in architecture 20, 61, 117–18, 125, 128, 130–1, 144, 147
　bird nest 130, 144
Swift, Jonathan 10

Tarlow, Sarah 3
total institution 17, 52, 102, 137

traitment moral 9
Tuke, Samuel 9–10, 16–17, 34–9, 45–6, 54–6, 61, 75, 83, 93, 114, 121–8, 130, 133–5, 137, 146, 150, 153
　see also York Retreat
Tuke, William 35–7
　see also York Retreat

Van Gennep, Arnold 24–5, 71, 101, 139
　see also Rites of Passage, The
ventilation 45, 87, 115–16, 118, 122, 125–6, 152
Vision for Change, A 151

Wakefield Asylum *see* West Riding Asylum
Wales 10, 38, 51
Watson and Pritchett 39, 61–2, 79, 96, 100, 122, 124–6, 130–2, 134, 152
Watson, Charles *see* Watson and Pritchett
West Riding Asylum 12, 27, 36–7 39, 43–6, 48–9, 55–8, 61–4, 71, 79, 80–2, 85–6, 88–91, 93, 95–6, 100, 104, 106–7 109–10, 112–13, 121–7, 130, 132, 134–7, 139, 140–1, 144, 152
asylums of the West Riding 89
Wexford County Lunatic Asylum 1
Whitworth Surgical Hospital 134, 142
Wide Streets Commission improvements 6, 52, 80
Willis, Francis 35, 38
workhouses xii, 4, 5, 7–8, 10, 13, 16, 18–19, 21, 32–3, 52, 55, 65–6, 73–4, 81–2, 87–8, 97, 99–100, 106–8, 116–19, 121, 138, 141–2, 144, 147, 155

York County Asylum 35
York Retreat 9, 16, 35–8, 55, 119, 121, 133–5, 146

EU authorised representative for GPSR:
Easy Access System Europe, Mustamäe tee 50,
10621 Tallinn, Estonia
gpsr.requests@easproject.com

www.ingramcontent.com/pod-product-compliance
Ingram Content Group UK Ltd.
Pitfield, Milton Keynes, MK11 3LW, UK
UKHW021828210426
5322IPUK00003B/69